HIV ESSENTIALS

Second Edition

Paul E. Sax, MD
Clinical Director, Division of Infectious Diseases and HIV Program
Brigham and Women's Hospital
Associate Professor of Medicine
Harvard Medical School
Boston, MA

Coeditors

Calvin J. Cohen, MD, MS
Director of Research, Community Research Initiative of New England
Instructor of Medicine
Harvard Medical School
Boston, MA

Daniel R. Kuritzkes, MD
Director of AIDS Research
Brigham and Women's Hospital
Professor of Medicine
Harvard Medical School
Boston, MA

PHYSICIANS' PRESS
A DIVISION OF JONES AND BARTLETT PUBLISHERS
Sudbury, Massachusetts
BOSTON TORONTO LONDON SINGAPORE

World Headquarters
Jones and Bartlett
Publishers
40 Tall Pine Drive
Sudbury, MA 01776
978-443-5000
info@jbpub.com
www.jbpub.com

Jones and Bartlett
Publishers Canada
6339 Ormindale Way
Mississauga, ON L5V 1J2
CANADA

Jones and Bartlett
Publishers International
Barb House, Barb Mews
London W6 7PA
UK

Jones and Bartlett's books and products are available through most bookstores and online booksellers. To contact Jones and Bartlett Publishers directly, call 800-832-0034, fax 978-443-8000, or visit our website at www.jbpub.com.

Substantial discounts on bulk quantities of Jones and Bartlett's publications are available to corporations, professional associations, and other qualified organizations. For details and specific discount information, contact the special sales department at Jones and Bartlett via the above contact information or send an email to specialsales@jbpub.com.

6048

ISBN-13: 978-0-7637-6124-0

Printed in the United States of America
12 11 10 09 08 10 9 8 7 6 5 4 3 2 1

EDITORIAL NOTE

This revised edition of HIV Essentials comes after an extraordinary phase in HIV drug development. Since the release of our inaugural edition last year, three new antiretroviral agents (maraviroc, raltegravir, and etravirine) have been approved by the FDA. These agents – usually used in combination with the newer protease inhibitors darunavir or tipranavir – bring to patients with drug-resistant HIV the opportunity to achieve virologic suppression at rates previously seen only in treatment-naive individuals. As a result, many such patients are achieving undetectable levels of HIV RNA for the first time in their life. Follow-up data on these exciting drugs suggest that these responses will be durable. As a result, the treatment goal for treatment-experienced patients is now the same as those starting therapy for the first time – that is, an HIV RNA below the limits of detection using the most sensitive assays (< 50-75 copies/mL).

With this progress in treatment, however, comes further complexity. The goal of this guide is to provide practitioners actively involved in HIV care with rapid access to practical information useful for patient management. When possible, we have cited US national guidelines from the Department of Health and Human Services; these are available at aidsinfo.nih.gov, and readers are advised to check this site for the most recent updates. We have also provided recommendations based on our interpretation of clinical trials, cohort studies, case reports, and personal experience.

This volume is dedicated to people living with HIV who have partnered with us to learn how to manage this condition, and to the doctors, nurses, social workers, pharmacists, and other health care professionals who focus on HIV as a specialty and continue to teach us how to get better at what we do.

Paul E. Sax, MD
Calvin J. Cohen, MD
Daniel R. Kuritzkes, MD

TABLES AND FIGURES

TABLE OF CONTENTS

CONTRIBUTORS

Paul E. Sax, MD
Clinical Director, Division of Infectious Diseases and HIV Program
Brigham and Women's Hospital
Associate Professor of Medicine
Harvard Medical School
Boston, Massachusetts

Calvin J. Cohen, MD, MS
Director of Research, Community Research Initiative of New England
Instructor of Medicine
Harvard Medical School
Boston, Massachusetts

Daniel R. Kuritzkes, MD
Director of AIDS Research
Brigham and Women's Hospital
Associate Professor of Medicine
Harvard Medical School
Boston, Massachusetts

Burke A. Cunha, MD,
Chief, Infectious Disease Division
Winthrop-University Hospital
Mineola, New York
Professor of Medicine
SUNY School of Medicine
Stony Brook, New York

Mark S. Freed, MD
President and Editor-in-Chief
Physicians' Press
Royal Oak, Michigan

David W. Kubiak, PharmD, BCPS
Infectious Disease Clinical Pharmacist
Brigham and Women's Hospital
Adjunct Clinical Assistant Professor of Pharmacy
Bouvé College of Health Sciences
School of Pharmacy
Northeastern University
Boston, Massachusetts

Damary C. Torres, PharmD
Clinical Pharmacy Specialist
Winthrop-University Hospital
Mineola, New York
Associate Clinical Professor of Pharmacy, College of Pharmacy
St. John's University
Queens, New York

Athe Tsibris, MD
Instructor in Medicine
Harvard Medical School
Massachusetts General Hospital
Boston, Massachusetts

Ruth Tuomala, MD
Director of Ob/Gyn Infectious Diseases
Brigham and Women's Hospital
Assistant Professor of Obstetrics, Gynecology, and Reproductive Biology
Harvard Medical School
Boston, Massachusetts

ACKNOWLEDGMENTS

To accomplish the task of presenting the data compiled in this reference, a small, dedicated team of professionals was assembled. This team focused their energy and discipline for many months into typing, revising, designing, illustrating, and formatting the many chapters that make up this text. We wish to acknowledge Monica Crowder Kaufman for her important contribution. We would also like to thank the many contributors who graciously contributed their time and energy, and Mark Freed, MD, President and Editor-in-Chief of Physicians' Press, for his vision, commitment, and guidance.

Paul E. Sax, MD
Calvin J. Cohen, MD
Daniel R. Kuritzkes, MD

NOTICE

ABBREVIATIONS FOR ANTIRETROVIRAL AGENTS

3TC lamivudine
ABC abacavir
ATV atazanavir
d4T stavudine
ddC zalcitabine
ddI didanosine
DLV delavirdine
DRV darunavir
EFV efavirenz
ETR etravirine
FPV fosamprenavir
FTC emtricitabine
IDV indinavir
LPV/r lopinavir/ritonavir
MVC maraviroc
NFV nelfinavir
NVP nevirapine
RAL raltegravir
RTV ritonavir
SQV saquinavir
T-20 enfuvirtide
TDF tenofovir disoproxil fumarate
TPV tipranavir
ZDV zidovudine

OTHER ABBREVIATIONS

AFB acid fast bacilli
ALT alanine transferase
ANC absolute neutrophil count
ARC AIDS-related complex
ARDS adult respiratory distress syndrome
ART antiretroviral therapy
AST aspartamine transferase
β-lactams penicillins, cephalosporins, cephamycins (not monobactams or carbapenems)
BAL bronchoalveolar lavage
BID twice daily
CCU critical care unit
CD4 CD4 T-cell lymphocyte
CIE counter-immunoelectrophoresis
CMV cytomegalovirus
CNS central nervous system
CPK creatine phosphokinase
CrCl creatinine clearance
CSF cerebrospinal fluid
CT computerized tomography
DFA direct fluorescent antibody
DIC disseminated intravascular coagulation
DNA deoxyribonucleic acid
DS double strength
e.g. for example
ELISA enzyme-linked immunosorbent assay
EMB ethambutol
ENT ear, nose, throat
Enterobacteriaceae: Citrobacter, Edwardsiella, Enterobacter, E. coli, Klebsiella, Proteus, Providencia, Salmonella, Serratia, Shigella
ESR erythrocyte sedimentation rate
ESRD end-stage renal disease
ET endotracheal
FUO fever of unknown origin
GI gastrointestinal
gm gram
GU genitourinary

OTHER ABBREVIATIONS (cont'd)

HSV herpes simplex virus
HU hydroxyurea
I & D incision and drainage
IFA immunofluorescent antibody
IgA immunoglobulin A
IgG immunoglobulin G
IgM immunoglobulin M
IM intramuscular
INH isoniazid
IRIS immune reconstitution inflammatory syndrome
IV/PO IV or PO
IV intravenous
kg kilogram
L liter
LFT liver function test
MAC *Mycobacterium avium* complex
mcg microgram
mcL microliter
mg milligram
mL milliliter
min minute
MRI magnetic resonance imaging
MRSA methicillin-resistant *S. aureus*
MSSA methicillin-sensitive *S. aureus*
NNRTI non-nucleoside reverse transcriptase inhibitor
NRTI nucleoside reverse transcriptase inhibitor
NSAID nonsteroidal anti-inflammatory drug
OI opportunistic infection
PBS protected brush specimen
PCP *Pneumocystis jiroveci* (carinii) pneumonia
PCR polymerase chain reaction
PI protease inhibitor
PMN polymorphonuclear leucocytes
PPD purified protein derivative
PO oral
PZA pyrazinamide
q__h every __ hours
q__d every __ days
QD once daily
qmonth once a month
qweek once a week
RBC red blood cells
RBV ribavirin
RNA ribonucleic acid
RT-PCR reverse-transcriptase polymerase chain reaction
SGOT/SGPT serum transaminases
SLE systemic lupus erythematosus
sp. species
SQ subcutaneous
SS single strength
TB tuberculosis
TID three times per day
TMP trimethoprim
TMP-SMX trimethoprim-sulfamethoxazole
VCA viral capsid antigen
VZV varicella zoster virus
WBC white blood cells

Chapter 1

Overview of HIV Infection

OVERVIEW OF HIV INFECTION

Infection with Human Immunodeficiency Virus (HIV-1) leads to a chronic and without treatment usually fatal infection characterized by progressive immunodeficiency, a long clinical latency period, and opportunistic infections. The hallmark of HIV disease is infection and viral replication within T-lymphocytes expressing the CD4 antigen (helper-inducer lymphocytes), a critical component of normal cell-mediated immunity. Qualitative defects in CD4 responsiveness and progressive depletion in CD4 cell counts increase the risk for opportunistic infections such as *Pneumocystis jiroveci (carinii)* pneumonia, and neoplasms such as lymphoma and Kaposi's sarcoma. HIV infection can also disrupt blood monocyte, tissue macrophage, and B-lymphocyte (humoral immunity) function, predisposing to infection with encapsulated bacteria. Direct attack of CD4-positive cells in the central and peripheral nervous system can cause HIV meningitis, peripheral neuropathy, and dementia.

More than 1 million people in the United States and 30 million people worldwide are infected with HIV. Without treatment, the average time from acquisition of HIV to an AIDS-defining opportunistic infection is about 10 years; survival then averages 1-2 years. There is tremendous individual variability in these time intervals, with some patients progressing from acute HIV infection to death within 1-2 years, and others not manifesting HIV-related immunosuppression for > 20 years after HIV acquisition. Antiretroviral therapy and prophylaxis against opportunistic infections have markedly improved the overall prognosis of HIV disease. The approach to HIV infection is shown in Figure 1.1.

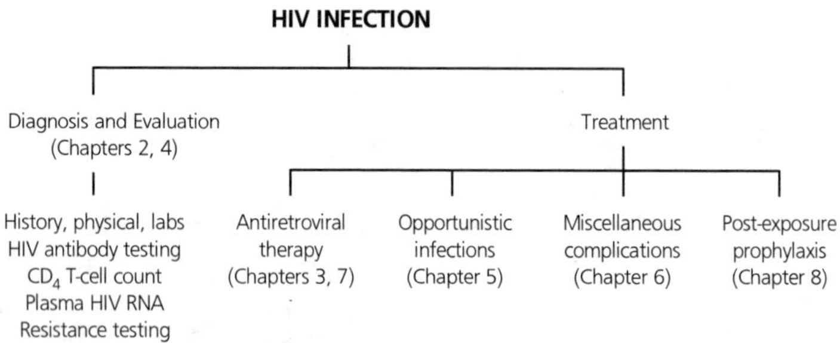

Figure 1.1. Approach to HIV Infection

STAGES OF HIV INFECTION

A. **Viral Transmission.** HIV infection is acquired primarily by sexual intercourse (anal, vaginal, infrequently oral), exposure to contaminated blood (primarily needle transmission), or maternal-fetus (perinatal) transmission. Sexual practices with the highest risk of transmission include unprotected receptive anal intercourse (especially with mucosal tearing), unprotected receptive vaginal intercourse (especially during menses), and unprotected rectal/vaginal intercourse in the presence of genital ulcers (e.g., primary syphilis, genital herpes, chancroid). Lower risk sexual practices include insertive anal/vaginal intercourse and oral-genital contact. The risk of transmission after a single encounter with an HIV source has been estimated to be 1 in 150 with needle sharing, 1 in 300 with occupational percutaneous exposure, 1 in 300-1000 with receptive anal intercourse, 1 in 500-1250 with receptive vaginal intercourse, 1 in 1000-3000 with insertive vaginal intercourse, and 1 in 3000 with insertive anal intercourse. Transmission risk increases with the number of encounters and with higher HIV RNA plasma levels. The mode of transmission does not affect the natural history of HIV disease, though patients with active or past injection drug use may have shortened survival due to comorbid complications.

B. **Acute (Primary) HIV Infection (pp. 8-9).** Acute HIV occurs 1-4 weeks after transmission, and is accompanied by a burst of viral replication with a decline in CD4 cell count. Most patients manifest a symptomatic mononucleosis-like syndrome, which is often overlooked. Acute HIV infection is confirmed by demonstrating a high HIV RNA in the absence of HIV antibody.

C. **Seroconversion.** Development of a positive HIV antibody test usually occurs within 4 weeks of acute infection, and invariably (with few exceptions) by 6 months.

D. **Asymptomatic HIV Infection** lasts a variable amount of time (average 8-10 years), and is accompanied by a gradual decline in CD4 cell counts and a relatively stable HIV RNA level (sometimes referred to as the viral "set point").

E. **Early Symptomatic HIV Infection.** Previously referred to as "AIDS Related Complex (ARC)," findings include thrush or vaginal candidiasis (persistent, frequent, or poorly responsive to treatment), herpes zoster (recurrent episodes or involving multiple dermatomes), oral hairy leukoplakia, peripheral neuropathy, diarrhea, or constitutional symptoms (e.g., low-grade fevers, weight loss).

F. **AIDS** is defined by a CD4 cell count $< 200/mm^3$, a CD4 cell percentage of total lymphocytes <14%, or one of several AIDS-related opportunistic infections. Common opportunistic infections include *Pneumocystis jiroveci (carinii)* pneumonia, cryptococcal meningitis, recurrent bacterial pneumonia, Candida esophagitis, CNS toxoplasmosis, tuberculosis, and non-Hodgkin's lymphoma. Other AIDS indicators in HIV-infected patients include candidiasis of the bronchi, trachea, or lungs; disseminated/extrapulmonary coccidiomycosis, cryptococcosis, or histoplasmosis; chronic (>1 month) intestinal cryptosporidiosis or isosporiasis; Kaposi's sarcoma; lymphoid interstitial pneumonia/pulmonary lymphoid hyperplasia; disseminated/extrapulmonary mycobacterial (non-tuberculous) infection; progressive multifocal leukoencephalopathy (PML); recurrent Salmonella septicemia; or HIV wasting syndrome.

G. **Advanced HIV Disease** corresponds with a CD4 cell count < 50/mm^3. Most AIDS-related deaths occur at this point. Common late stage opportunistic infections are caused by CMV disease (retinitis, colitis) or disseminated *Mycobacterium avium* complex (MAC).

ACUTE (PRIMARY) HIV INFECTION

A. **Description.** Acute clinical illness associated with primary acquisition of HIV, occurring 1-4 weeks after viral transmission (range: 6 days to 6 weeks). Symptoms develop in 50-90%, but are often mistaken for the flu, mononucleosis, or other nonspecific viral syndrome. More severe symptoms may correlate with a higher viral set point and more rapid HIV disease progression (J AIDS 2007;45:445-8). Even without therapy, most patients recover, reflecting development of a partially effective immune response and depletion of susceptible CD4 cells.

B. **Differential Diagnosis** includes **EBV, CMV**, viral hepatitis, enteroviral infection, 2° syphilis, toxoplasmosis, HSV with erythema multiforme, drug reaction, Behcet's disease, acute lupus.

C. **Signs and Symptoms** usually reflect hematogenous dissemination of virus to lymphoreticular and neurologic sites (N Engl J Med 1998;339:33-9):
- Fever (97%)
- Pharyngitis (73%). Typically non-exudative (unlike EBV, which is usually exudative)
- Rash (77%). Maculopapular viral exanthem of the face and trunk is most common, but can involve the extremities, palms and soles
- Arthralgia/myalgia (58%)
- Neurologic symptoms (12%). Headache is most common. Neuropathy, Bell's palsy, and meningoencephalitis are rare, but may predict worse outcome
- Oral/genital ulcerations, thrush, nausea, vomiting, diarrhea, weight loss

D. Laboratory Findings

1. **CBC.** Lymphopenia followed by lymphocytosis (common). Atypical lymphocytosis is variable, but usually low level (unlike EBV, where atypical lymphocytosis may be 20-30% or higher). Thrombocytopenia occurs in some.
2. **Elevated Transaminases** in some but not all patients.
3. **Depressed CD4 Cell Count.** Can rarely be low enough to induce opportunistic infections.
4. **HIV Antibody.** Usually negative, although persons with prolonged symptoms of acute HIV may have positive antibody tests if diagnosed late during the course of illness.

E. Confirming the Diagnosis of Acute HIV Infection

1. **Obtain HIV Antibody** after informed consent (if required by state law) to exclude prior disease
2. **Order Viral Load Test (HIV RNA PCR),** preferably RT-PCR. HIV RNA confirms acute HIV infection prior to seroconversion. Most individuals will have very high HIV RNA (> 100,000 copies/mL). Be suspicious of a false-positive test if the HIV RNA is low (< 10,000 copies/mL) (J Infect Dis 2004;190:598-604). For any positive test, it is important to repeat HIV RNA and HIV antibody testing. p24 antigen can also be used to establish the diagnosis, but is less sensitive than HIV RNA PCR.
3. **Order Other Tests/Serologies if HIV RNA Test is Negative.** Order throat cultures for bacterial/viral respiratory pathogens, EBV VCA IgM/IgG, CMV IgM/IgG, HHV-6 IgM/IgG, and hepatitis serologies as appropriate to establish a diagnosis for patient's symptoms.

F. Management of Acute HIV Infection

1. **Initiate Antiretroviral Therapy.** Patients with acute HIV infection should be referred to an HIV specialist, who ideally will enroll the patient into a clinical study. Many experts recommend antiretroviral therapy, although no long-term clinical studies comparing treatment vs. observation have been conducted. The optimal duration of therapy and role of intermittent treatment are under investigation. Regimens for treatment are similar to those outlined for chronic HIV infection (Table 3.2). Some clinicians elect to start with PI-based treatment given the risk of transmitted NNRTI resistance.
2. **Obtain HIV Resistance Genotype (Chapter 4)** because of the background prevalence of transmission of antiretroviral therapy-resistant virus. A genotype resistance test is preferred; therapy can be started pending results of the test.
3. **Rationale for Treatment of Acute HIV Infection.** No prospective clinical studies have conclusively documented the benefits of therapy for acute HIV infection. Possible benefits include hastening symptom resolution, reducing viral transmission, lowering virologic "set point," and preserving virus-specific CD4 responses. Eradication of HIV is not possible with currently available agents.

Chapter 2

Diagnosis and Evaluation of HIV Infection

HIV ANTIBODY TESTING

A. Standard HIV Antibody Tests (see also Clin Infect Dis 2007;45:S221-S225). HIV antibody tests (ELISA, Western blot) and quantitative plasma HIV RNA (HIV viral load) assays are used to diagnose HIV infection (Figure 2.1). Most patients produce antibody to HIV within 6-8 weeks of exposure; 50% will have a positive antibody test by 3-4 weeks, and nearly 100% will have detectable antibody by 6 months.

1. **ELISA.** Usual screening test. All positives are routinely confirmed with Western blot or other more specific tests.
2. **Western Blot.** CDC criteria for interpretation:
   a. **Positive.** At least two of the following bands present: p24, gp41, gp160/120
   b. **Negative.** No bands present
   c. **Indeterminate.** HIV band present, but does not meet criteria for positivity
3. **Test Performance.** Standard method is ELISA screen with Western blot confirmation.
   a. **ELISA negative.** Western blot is not required (ELISA sensitivity 99.7%, specificity 98.5%). Obtain HIV RNA if acute HIV infection is suspected.
   b. **ELISA positive.** Laboratories will confirm results with Western blot. Probability that ELISA and Western blot are both false-positives is extremely low (< 1 per 140,000). Absence of p31 band could be a clue to a false positive Western blot.
   c. **Unexpected ELISA/Western blot.** Repeat test to exclude clerical/computer error, the most common cause of incorrect results.
4. **Indeterminate Western Blot.** This occurs in approximately 4-20% of reactive ELISAs, usually due to a single p24 band or weak other bands. HIV-related causes include seroconversion in progress, advanced HIV disease with loss of antibody response, or infection with HIV-2. Non-HIV-related causes include cross-reacting antibody from pregnancy, blood transfusions, organ transplantation, autoantibodies from collagen vascular disease, influenza vaccination, or recipient of HIV vaccine. In low-risk patients, an indeterminate result rarely represents true HIV infection. Since seroconversion-in-progress is generally associated with high HIV RNA levels, the recommended approach is to obtain an HIV RNA test. In addition, most patients with indeterminate Western blots due to seroconversion-in-progress will develop a fully positive HIV test within one month.

B. Other HIV Antibody Tests

1. **Home Test Kit (Home Access HIV-1 Test System).** This system can be purchased over-the-counter at pharmacies, or ordered by phone or over the Internet (www.homeaccess.com). Users receive a kit that includes a stylet for obtaining a sample of blood from the fingertip, which is then placed on filter paper and mailed to the company for testing. The standard test will return a result within 7 days and costs $44; users can purchase overnight shipping for an additional cost and a more

rapid turnaround time. By using a code provided with each kit, users can call and obtain their results anonymously. Phone counseling is available to explain the results, as well as a database of local HIV providers if the test result is positive. The Home Access test employs ELISA testing, which is done in duplicate. All individuals with reactive tests on the system must have results confirmed by standard testing. As of 2008, there is no true home test that returns results to the user without the involvement of a central laboratory or health care facility; such tests are technically feasible and are being reviewed by the FDA.

2. **OraSure.** This office-based test was approved in 1996 and uses a special swab that collects oral mucosal transudate (not saliva) when it is held between the cheek and the gum. This system obtains quantities of antibody that are comparable to or exceed those from serum samples. Once the specimen is collected, it is sent to a central laboratory for ELISA and Western blot testing, which can be performed on the same sample. As a result, the sensitivity and specificity of the test are comparable to standard blood HIV antibody testing (JAMA 1997;277:254).
3. **Rapid HIV Test (OraQuick ADVANCE Rapid HIV Test).** This test was approved in 2004 and can be performed on whole blood, plasma, or oral mucosal transudate samples. Results are returned in 20 minutes and are comparable in accuracy to a single ELISA test. As a result, *a reactive rapid test must be confirmed with standard ELISA/Western blot serology*. A major advantage of this rapid test includes the ability to give patients a negative result at the time of care; there also is some evidence that individuals given a positive rapid test result are more likely to return for their confirmative serology results. Since the test can be done at the point of care (no CLIA certification is required), it is particularly useful in the evaluation of source patients of needlestick injuries and for women in labor who did not receive HIV testing during prenatal care.

C. Selected Other Licensed HIV Diagnostic Tests

1. **p24 Antigen.** Approved for diagnosis of acute HIV infection. However, due to low sensitivity of this test, HIV RNA has replaced p24 antigen in clinical practice, and hence this test is rarely ordered.
2. **Nucleic Acid Based Tests.** In the United States, donated blood has been screened with nucleic acid based tests since the late 1990s, shortening the time between infection and detectability of infection to about 12 days. As a result, the rate of acquiring HIV from a blood transfusion is now estimated at one infection per 2 million units transfused (JAMA 2003;289:959). A related test, the Aptima HIV-1 RNA Qualitative Assay, was approved for HIV diagnosis in 2006. Like quantitative HIV RNA tests, this assay can be used to diagnose acute HIV infection before antibodies develop, but results are provided only as positive or negative. Additionally, it can confirm HIV infection in a person with a positive HIV ELISA or rapid test. It is not known whether the rate of false positivity with the Aptima test is lower than the rate with RT-PCR or bDNA.

QUANTITATIVE PLASMA HIV RNA (HIV VIRAL LOAD ASSAYS)

HIV viral load assays measure the amount of HIV RNA in plasma. The high sensitivity of these assays allows detection of virus in most patients not on antiretroviral therapy. These test are used to diagnose acute HIV infection, and more commonly to monitor the response to antiretroviral therapy.

A. Uses of HIV RNA Assay

1. **Confirms Diagnosis of Acute HIV Infection.** A high HIV RNA with a negative HIV antibody test confirms acute HIV infection prior to seroconversion.
2. **Helpful in Initial Evaluation of HIV Infection.** Establishes baseline HIV RNA and helps (along with CD4 cell count) determine whether to initiate or defer therapy, as HIV RNA correlates with rate of CD4 decline.
3. **Monitors Response to Antiviral Therapy.** HIV RNA changes rapidly decline 2-4 weeks after starting or changing effective antiretroviral therapy, with slower decline thereafter. Patients with the greatest HIV RNA response have the best clinical outcome. No change in HIV RNA suggests that therapy will be ineffective or the patient is noncompliant.
4. **Estimates Risk for Opportunistic Infection.** For patients with similar CD4 cell counts, the risk of opportunistic infections is higher with higher HIV RNAs. HIV RNA is not formally incorporated into opportunistic infection prevention guidelines.

B. Assays and Interpretation

1. **Tests, Sensitivities, and Dynamic Range**. Several assays are used, each with advantages and disadvantages; most US sites use RT-PCR or bDNA. Any assay can be used to diagnose acute HIV infection and guide/monitor therapy, but the same test should be used to follow patients longitudinally.
   a. **RT-PCR Amplicor** (Roche): Sensitivity = 400 copies/mL; dynamic range = 400-750,000 copies/mL
   b. **RT-PCR Ultrasensitive 1.5** (Roche): Sensitivity = 50 copies/mL; dynamic range = 50-75,000 copies/mL
   c. **bDNA Versant 3.0** (Bayer): Sensitivity = 75 copies/mL; dynamic range = 75-500,000 copies/mL
   d. **Nucleic acid sequence-based amplification** (NASBA), NucliSens HIV-1 QT (bioMerieux). Sensitivity = 176 copies/mL; dynamic range = 176-3.5 million copies/mL (depends on volume)
   e. **Real Time HIV-1 assay** (Abbott)**:** PCR-based assay. Sensitivity = 40 copies/mL; dynamic range = 40-10 million copies/mL
   f. **COBAS AmpliPrep/COBAS TagMan HIV-1 test** (Roche): Sensitivity = 48 copies/mL; dynamic range = 48-10 million copies/mL

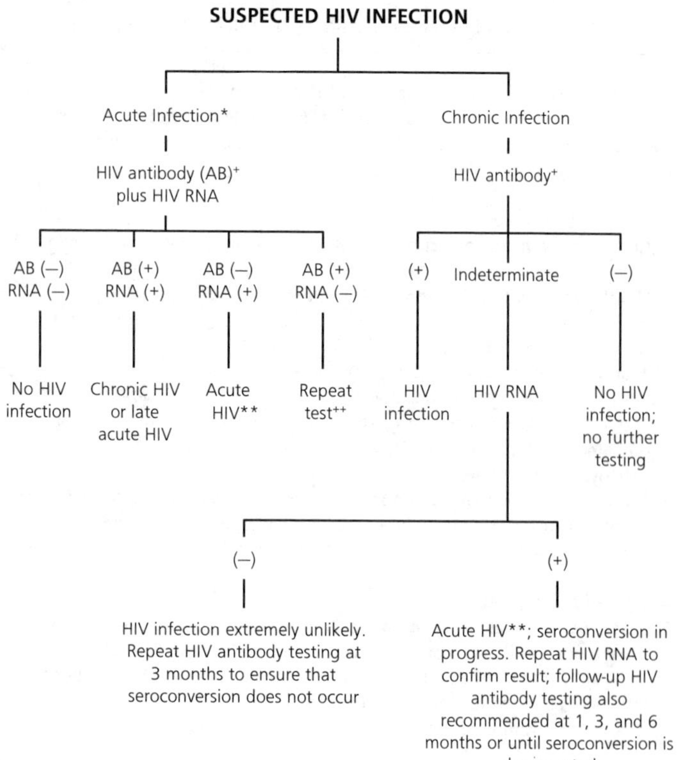

Figure 2.1. Approach to HIV Testing

(–) negative test; (+) positive test

* Occurs 1-4 weeks after viral transmission. Most patients manifest a viral syndrome (fever, pharyngitis ± rash/arthralgias), which is often mistaken for mononucleosis or the flu and therefore overlooked

** HIV RNA in acute HIV infection should be very high (usually > 100,000 copies/mL)

\+ All positive ELISA tests must be confirmed by Western Blot; usually this is done automatically in clinical laboratories

++ May be long-term non-progressor or laboratory error

2. **Correlation Between HIV RNA and CD4 Cell Count.** HIV RNA assays correlate inversely with CD4 cell counts, but do so imperfectly (e.g., some patients with high CD4 counts have relatively high HIV RNA levels, and vice versa.) For any given CD4, higher HIV RNA levels correlate with more rapid CD4 decline. In response to antiretroviral therapy, changes in HIV RNA generally precede changes in CD4 cell count.
3. **Significant Change in HIV RNA Assay.** This is defined by at least a 2-fold (0.3 log) change in viral RNA (accounts for normal variation in clinically stable patients), or a 3-fold (0.5 log) change in response to new antiretroviral therapy (accounts for intra-laboratory and patient variability). For example, if a HIV RNA result = 50,000 copies/mL, then the range of possible actual values = 25,000-100,000 copies/mL, and the value needed to demonstrate antiretroviral activity is ≤ 17,000 copies/mL.

C. **Indications for HIV RNA Testing**. This test is usually performed in conjunction with CD4 cell counts, and is indicated for the diagnosis of acute HIV infection and for initial evaluation of newly diagnosed HIV. It is also recommended 2-8 weeks after initiation of antiretroviral therapy and every 3-4 months in all HIV patients.

D. **When to Avoid HIV RNA Testing**

1. **During Acute Illnesses and Immunizations.** Patients with acute infections (opportunistic infection, bacterial pneumonia, even HSV recurrences) may experience significant (> 5-fold) rises in HIV RNA, which return to baseline 1-2 months after recovery. Although data are conflicting, many studies show at least a transient increase in HIV RNA levels following influenza and other immunizations, which return to baseline after 1-2 months.
2. **When Test Results Would Not Influence Therapy.** This is a frequent scenario in patients with advanced disease who have no antiretroviral options or cannot tolerate therapy.
3. **As a Screening Test for HIV Infection,** except if acute (primary) HIV disease is suspected during the HIV antibody window (i.e., first 3-6 weeks after viral transmission). HIV RNA tests have an unacceptably high false-positive rate when used for this purpose (J Infect Dis 2004;190:598-604).

INITIAL ASSESSMENT OF HIV-INFECTED PATIENTS

A. **Clinical Evaluation.** The history and physical examination should focus on diagnoses associated with HIV infection. Compared to patients without HIV, the severity, frequency, and duration of these conditions are usually increased in HIV disease.

1. **Dermatologic:** Severe herpes simplex (oral/anogenital); herpes zoster (especially recurrent, cranial nerve, or disseminated); molluscum contagiosum; staphylococcal

abscesses; tinea nail infections; Kaposi's sarcoma (from HHV-8 infection); petechiae (from ITP); seborrheic dermatitis; new or worsening psoriasis; eosinophilic pustular folliculitis; severe cutaneous drug eruptions (especially sulfonamides)

2. **Oropharyngeal:** Oral candidiasis; oral hairy leukoplakia (from EBV); Kaposi's sarcoma (most commonly on palate or gums); gingivitis/periodontitis; warts; aphthous ulcers (especially esophageal/perianal)
3. **Constitutional symptoms:** Fatigue, fevers, chronic diarrhea, weight loss
4. **Lymphatic:** Persistent, generalized lymphadenopathy
5. **Others:** Active TB (especially extrapulmonary); non-Hodgkin's lymphoma (especially CNS); unexplained leukopenia, anemia, thrombocytopenia (especially ITP); myopathy; miscellaneous neurologic conditions (cranial/peripheral neuropathies, Guillain-Barre syndrome, mononeuritis multiplex, aseptic meningitis, cognitive impairment)

B. Baseline Laboratory Testing (Table 2.1) (See also Clin Infect Disease 2004;39:609-29).

C. CD4 Cell Count (Lymphocyte Subset Analysis)

Table 2.1. Baseline Laboratory Testing for HIV-Infected Patients*

Test	Rationale
Repeat HIV serology (ELISA/confirmatory Western blot)	Indicated for patients unable to document a prior positive test, and for "low risk" individuals with a positive test (to detect computer/clerical error). Repeat serology is now less important since HIV RNA testing provides an additional means of confirming HIV infection. Also useful in ruling out cases of suspected factitious HIV
CBC with differential, platelets	Detects cytopenias (e.g., ITP) seen in HIV. Needed to calculate CD4 cell count
Chemistry panel ("SMA 20")	Detects renal dysfunction and electrolyte/LFT/glucose abnormalities, which may accompany HIV and associated infections (e.g., HIV nephropathy, HCV)
Fasting lipid profile	Since HIV and many antiretroviral agents influence lipid levels, a lipid profile before treatment provides a useful baseline
CD4 cell count	Determines the need for antiretroviral therapy and opportunistic infection (OI) prophylaxis. Best test for defining risk of OI's and prognosis
HIV RNA assay ("viral load")	Provides a marker for the pace of HIV disease progression. Determines indication for and response to antiretroviral therapy
HIV resistance genotype	Identifies patients infected with a resistant virus (some resistance now detected in approximately 15% of newly diagnosed patients in the US)

Table 2.1. Baseline Laboratory Testing for HIV-Infected Patients*

Test	Rationale
Tuberculin skin test (standard 5 TU of PPD)	Detects latent TB infection and targets patients for preventive therapy. Anergy skin tests are not recommended due to poor predictive value. HIV is the most powerful co-factor for the development of active TB
PAP smear	Risk of cervical cancer is nearly twice as high in HIV-positive women vs. uninfected controls; some advocate anal pap smears for gay men
Toxoplasmosis serology (IgG)	Identifies patients at risk for subsequent cerebral/systemic toxoplasmosis and the need for prophylaxis. Those with negative tests should be counseled on how to avoid infection
Syphilis serology (VDRL or RPR)	Identifies co-infection with syphilis, which is epidemiologically-linked to HIV. Disease may have accelerated course in HIV patients
Hepatitis C serology (anti-HCV)	Identifies HCV infection and usually chronic carriage. If positive, follow with HCV genotype and HCV viral load assay. If patient is antibody-negative but at high-risk for hepatitis, order HCV RNA to exclude a false-negative result
Hepatitis B serologies (HBsAb, HBcAb, HBsAg)	Identifies patients who are immune to hepatitis B (HBsAb) or chronic carriers (HBsAg). If all three are negative, hepatitis B vaccine is indicated
Hepatitis A serology (anti-HAV)	Identifies candidates for hepatitis A vaccine; if anti-HAV positive, already immune
G6PD screen	Identifies patients at risk for dapsone or primaquine-associated hemolysis
CMV serology (IgG)	Identifies patients who should receive CMV-negative or leukocyte-depleted blood if transfused
VZV serology (IgG)	Identifies patients at risk for varicella (chickenpox), and those who should avoid contact with active varicella or herpes zoster patients. Serology-negative patients exposed to chickenpox should receive varicella-zoster immune globulin (VZIG); some advocate varicella vaccine if CD4 > $350/mm^3$
Chest x-ray	Sometimes ordered as a baseline test for future comparisons. May detect healed granulomatous diseases/other processes. Indicated in all tuberculin skin test positive patients
HLA-B*5701	Needed if therapy with abacavir is planned. Patients negative for HLA-B*5701 have almost no risk of severe hypersensitivity reaction to abacavir

* See also Clin Infect Dis 2004;39:609-29

Table 2.2. Use of CD4 Cell Count for Interpretation of Patient Signs and Symptoms in HIV Infection

CD4 (cells/mm^3)	Associated Conditions
> 500	Most illnesses are similar to those in HIV-negative patients. Some increased risk of bacterial infections (pneumococcal pneumonia, sinusitis), herpes zoster, tuberculosis, skin conditions
200-500*	Bacterial infections (especially pneumococcal pneumonia, sinusitis), cutaneous Kaposi's sarcoma, vaginal candidiasis, ITP
50-200*	Thrush, oral hairy leukoplakia, classic HIV-associated opportunistic infections (e.g., *P. jiroveci [carinii]* pneumonia, cryptococcal meningitis, toxoplasmosis). For patients receiving prophylaxis, most opportunistic infection do not occur until CD4 cell counts < 100/mm^3 (Ann Intern Med 1996;124:633-42)
< 50*	"Final common pathway" opportunistic infections (disseminated *M. avium* complex, CMV retinitis), HIV-associated wasting, neurologic disease (neuropathy, encephalopathy)

* Patients remain at risk for all processes noted in earlier stages

1. **Overview.** Acute HIV infection is characterized by a decline in CD4 cell count, followed by a gradual rise associated with clinical recovery. Chronic HIV infection shows progressive declines (~ 50-80 cells/year, but with wide interpatient variability) in CD4 cell count without treatment, followed by more rapid decline 1-2 years prior to opportunistic infection(AIDS-defining diagnosis). Cell counts remain stable over 5-10 years in 5% of patients, while others may show rapid declines (> 300 cells/year). Since variability exists within individual patients and between laboratories, it is useful to *repeat any value before making management decisions.*
2. **Uses of CD4 Cell Count**
   a. **Gives context of degree of immunosuppression** for interpretation of symptoms/signs (Table 2.2)
   b. **Used to guide therapy.** Guidelines support CD4 cell counts < 200/mm^3 as a key threshold before which treatment should be initiated, regardless of HIV RNA or symptoms; treatment should be strongly considered for CD4 < 200-350. For prophylaxis against PCP, toxoplasmosis, and MAC/CMV infection, CD4 cell counts of 200/mm^3, < 100/mm^3, and < 50/mm^3 are used as threshold levels, respectively
   c. **Provides estimate of risk of opportunistic infection or death.** CD4 cell counts < 50/mm^3 are associated with a markedly increased risk of death (median survival 1 year without treatment), although some patients with low counts survive > 3 years even without antiretroviral therapy. Prognosis is heavily influenced by HIV RNA, presence/history of opportunistic infections or neoplasms, performance status, and the immunologic response to antiretroviral therapy

Chapter 3

Treatment of HIV Infection

INITIATION OF ANTIRETROVIRAL THERAPY (Figure 3.1)

Combination antiretroviral therapy has led to dramatic reductions in HIV-related morbidity and mortality for patients with severe immunosuppression (CD4 < 200 cells/mm^3) or a prior AIDS-defining illness. Treatment of asymptomatic patients is far also now recommended for those with CD4 cell counts between 200-350 cells/mm^3. Potential benefits of starting antiretroviral therapy with relatively high CD4 cell counts include reduction in HIV RNA, prevention of immunodeficiency, delayed time to onset of AIDS, and decreased risk of drug toxicity, viral transmission, and selecting resistant virus. Potential risks of early antiretroviral therapy include reduced quality of life (from side effects/inconvenience), earlier development of drug resistance (with consequent transmission of resistant virus), limitation in future antiretroviral choices, unknown long-term toxicity of antiretroviral drugs, and unknown duration of effectiveness.

The primary goals of therapy are prolonged suppression of viral replication to undetectable levels (HIV RNA < 50-75 copies/mL), restoration/preservation of immune function, and improved clinical outcome. Once initiated, antiretroviral therapy should be continued indefinitely. One possible exception is when treatment is started in pregnant women with CD4 cell counts > 350 solely to reduce the risk of maternal-child transmission. Such women may have treatment stopped after delivery, based on patient and clinician preference.

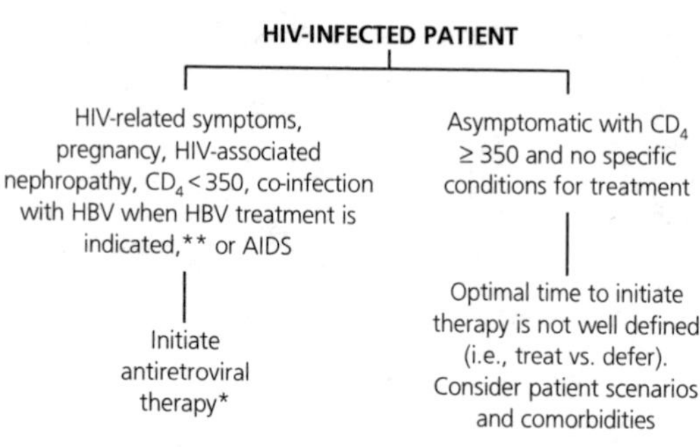
HIV-INFECTED PATIENT
HIV-related symptoms, pregnancy, HIV-associated nephropathy, CD_4 < 350, co-infection with HBV when HBV treatment is indicated,** or AIDS
Initiate antiretroviral therapy*
Asymptomatic with CD_4 ≥ 350 and no specific conditions for treatment
Optimal time to initiate therapy is not well defined (i.e., treat vs. defer). Consider patient scenarios and comorbidities

Figure 3.1. Indications for Initiating Antiretroviral Therapy

* See Tables 3.3 and 3.4

** Treat with fully suppressive antiviral drugs active against both HIV and hepatitis B virus (HBV)

Adapted from: Guidelines for the Use of Antiretroviral Agents for HIV-1-infected Adults and Adolescents: recommendations of the Panel on Clinical Practices for Treatment of HIV Infection; www.hivatis.org, January 29, 2008

Table 3.1. Antiretroviral Agents Used for HIV Infection

Drug (abbreviation; trade name, manufacturer)	Formulations	Usual Adult Dosing§	Comments
NUCLEOSIDE (AND NUCLEOTIDE) REVERSE TRANSCRIPTASE INHIBITORS (NRTI's)			
Abacavir sulfate (ABC; Ziagen, GlaxoSmithKline)	300-mg tablets; 20-mg/mL oral solution	300 mg bid or 600 mg qd	Pretreatment screening for HLA-B*5701 is recommended. No clinically significant drug interactions documented. Do not use in patients with a history of abacavir hypersensitivity reaction. Avoid in patients with moderate-severe hepatic impairment. Treatment may be associated with increased risk of MI (Lancet 2008; April 1, e-pub)
Abacavir sulfate/lamivudine (Epzicom, GlaxoSmithKline)	600/300-mg tablet	One 600/300 mg tablet qd	See abacavir and lamivudine
Abacavir sulfate/ lamivudine/zidovudine (Trizivir, GlaxoSmithKline)	300/150/300-mg tablet	One 300/150/300 mg tablet bid	See abacavir, lamivudine, zidovudine
Didanosine (ddI; Videx/Videx EC, Bristol-Myers Squibb; Oncology/Immunology; also available generically)	125-, 200-, 250-, 400-mg delayed-release enteric-coated capsules; 100-, 167-, 250-mg powder	Capsule: < 60 kg: 250 mg qd ≥ 60 kg: 400 mg qd 250 mg qd with tenofovir (best avoided) Powder: < 60 kg: 167 mg bid ≥ 60 kg: 250 mg bid probably Administration: Take on empty stomach at least 30 minutes before or 2 hours after meal	Avoid concomitant ribavirin use due to drug-drug interaction that increases ddI toxicity. If possible, avoid concomitant tenofovir due to impaired CD4 response and increased risk of virologic failure in treatment naive patients. Treatment may be associated with increased risk of MI (Lancet 2008; April 1, e-pub)

Table 3.1. Antiretroviral Agents Used for HIV Infection (cont'd)

Drug (abbreviation; trade name, manufacturer)	Formulations	Usual Adult Dosing§	Comments
NUCLEOSIDE (AND NUCLEOTIDE) REVERSE TRANSCRIPTASE INHIBITORS (NRTI's) (cont'd)			
Emtricitabine (FTC; Emtriva, Gilead Sciences)	200-mg capsule	200 mg qd	No clinically significant drug interactions. Exacerbations of HBV reported in patients coinfected with HIV and HBV after discontinuation of emtricitabine
Lamivudine (3TC; Epivir, GlaxoSmithKline)	150-, 300-mg tablets; 10-mg/mL oral solution	150 mg bid or 300 mg qd	No clinically significant drug interactions. Exacerbations of HBV reported in patients coinfected with HIV and HBV after discontinuation of lamivudine
Lamivudine/zidovudine (Combivir, GlaxoSmithKline)	150/300-mg tablet	One 150/300-mg tablet bid	See zidovudine and lamivudine
Stavudine (d4T; Zerit, Bristol-Myers Squibb Virology)	15-, 20-, 30-, 40-mg capsules; 1-mg/mL oral solution	< 60 kg: 30 mg bid ≥ 60 kg: 40 mg bid	Do not coadminister with didanosine due to increased risk of lipoatrophy and peripheral neuropathy. Antagonistic with zidovudine; do not coadminister
Tenofovir disoproxil fumarate (TDF; Viread, Gilead Sciences)	300-mg tablet	One 300-mg tablet qd	Dosing interval adjustment is recommended in all patients with CrCl < 50 mL/min. Lowers levels of atazanavir; ritonavir boosting of atazanavir is required. Avoid concomitant didanosine due to impaired CD4 response and increased risk of virologic failure
Tenofovir disoproxil fumarate/emtricitabine (Truvada, Gilead Sciences)	300/200-mg tablet	One 300/200-mg tablet qd	Dose adjustment required for CrCl < 50 mL/min
Zidovudine (ZDV; Retrovir, GlaxoSmithKline; also available generically)	100-mg capsule; 300-mg tablet; 10-mg/5 mL oral solution; 10-mg/mL IV solution	200 mg tid or 300 mg bid (or with 3TC as Combivir or with abacavir and 3TC as Trizivir) 5-6 mg/kg daily	Hematologic side effects more common with advanced HIV disease (CD4 < 200/mm^3)

Table 3.1. Antiretroviral Agents Used for HIV Infection (cont'd)

Drug (abbreviation; trade name, manufacturer)	Formulations	Usual Adult Dosing§	Comments
NON-NUCLEOSIDE REVERSE TRANSCRIPTASE INHIBITORS (NNRTI's)*			
Delavirdine mesylate (DLV; Rescriptor, Agouron)‡	100-, 200-mg tablets	400 mg tid (100-mg tablets can be dispersed in water; 200-mg tablet should be taken intact). Separate dosing from ddI or antacids by 1 hour, with or without food	Rash, if not severe, is often treatable with antihistamines and corticosteroids
Efavirenz (EFV; Sustiva, Bristol-Myers Squibb Oncology/ Immunology; outside USA known as Stocrin)‡	50-, 100-, 200-mg capsules; 600-mg tablet	600 mg qd; best taken prior to bed due reduce incidence of CNS side effects	CNS side effects usually resolve after 1-2 weeks. Rash, if not severe, is often treatable with antihistamines and corticosteroids. Contraindicated during pregnancy (category rating "D"); use with caution in women of childbearing potential and advise on use
Etravirine (ETR; Intelence, Tibotec Therapeutics)	100 mg tablets	Two 100-mg tablets after a meal	Indicated for patients with prior treatment failure on NNRTI-based therapy. Rash occurs in approximately 16% of recipients, generally in week two of therapy. If mild, can continue therapy and rash will usually resolve
Nevirapine (NVP; Viramune, Boehringer Ingelheim)‡	200-mg tablet; 50-mg/5 mL oral suspension (pediatric)	200 mg qd x 2 weeks, then 200 mg bid	Risk of hypersensitivity (hepatitis, skin rash) increased for men with CD4 > 400/mm^3, and women > 250/mm^3; avoid use in these patients unless benefit outweighs risk
COMBINATION NRTI/NNRTI			
Efavirenz/emtricitabine/ tenofovir (Atripla, Bristol-Myers Squibb & Gilead)	600/200/300-mg tablet	One 600/200/300-mg tablet daily	See efavirenz, emtricitabine, tenofovir

Table 3.1. Antiretroviral Agents Used for HIV Infection (cont'd)

Drug (abbreviation; trade name, manufacturer)	Formulations	Usual Adult Dosing§	Comments
	PROTEASE INHIBITORS (PI's)†		
Atazanavir sulfate (ATV; Reyataz, Bristol-Myers Squibb Virology)‡	100-, 150-, 200-, 300-mg capsules	400 mg qd, or 300 mg qd in combination with ritonavir 100 mg qd. For treatment-experienced patients, or when used with tenofovir or efavirenz or nevirapine use: 300 mg in combination with 100 mg of ritonavir. Take with food	Indirect hyperbilirubinemia; rarely severe enough to lead to drug discontinuation. Gastric acidity required for absorption (proton pump-inhibitors contraindicated). May give atazanavir 2 or more hours before or 10 hours after H_2 blockers
Fosamprenavir (FPV; Lexiva, GlaxoSmithKline)‡	700-mg tablet	PI-naïve patients: 1400 mg bid, or 700 mg bid in combination with ritonavir 100 mg bid, or 1400 mg qd in combination with ritonavir 200 mg qd or 100 mg qd PI-experienced patients: 700 mg bid in combination with ritonavir 100 mg bid	Reduces levels of several other PI's; coadministration not recommended
Indinavir sulfate (IDV; Crixivan, Merck)‡	200-, 333-, 400-mg capsules	800 mg tid, or 800 mg bid in combination with ritonavir 100 mg or 200 mg bid Administration: *Unboosted*: Take 1 hour before or 2 hours after meals; may take with skim milk/low-fat meal. *Boosted*: Take with or without food. Separate dosing from ddI by 1 hour	Instruct patients to drink 6-8 glasses of water per day to reduce risk of nephrolithiasis

Table 3.1. Antiretroviral Agents Used for HIV Infection (cont'd)

Drug (abbreviation; trade name, manufacturer)	Formulations	Usual Adult Dosing§	Comments
	PROTEASE INHIBITORS (PI's)† (cont'd)		
Lopinavir/ritonavir (LPV/r; Kaletra, Abbott)‡	200/50 mg tablet; 80/20-mg/mL oral solution	Two tablets (400/100 mg) bid; 5 mL oral solution bid. Four tablets (800/200 mg) qd an option for treatment-naive patients. With EFV or NVP: 3 tablets (600/150 mg) bid or 6.7 mL bid	Oral solution contains 42.4% alcohol. Tablets may be taken with or without food
Nelfinavir mesylate (NFV; Viracept, Agouron/Pfizer)	250-, 625-mg tablets; 50-mg/gm oral powder	750 mg tid or 1250 mg bid. Take with food	Diarrhea can usually be controlled with antidiarrheals (loperamide, pectin)
Ritonavir (RTV; Norvir, Abbott)‡	100-mg capsule; 600 mg/7.5 mL solution; 80 mg/mL oral solution	600 mg bid as sole PI; 100-400 mg daily in 1-2 divided doses as pharmacokinetic booster for other PI's Administration: Take with food or up to 2 hours after a meal to improve tolerability	Used nearly exclusively as pharmacokinetic booster of other PI's
Saquinavir (SQV; Invirase, Roche)‡	200-, 500-mg hard-gel capsules	1000 mg bid in combination with ritonavir 100 mg bid. Take with food	Must be given with ritonavir boosting. Increased risk of hepatitis when rifampin dosed with saquinavir plus ritonavir. Saquinavir soft-gel capsules (Fortovase) no longer available
Tipranavir (TPV; Aptivus, Boehringer Ingelheim)‡	250-mg soft-gel capsule	500 mg bid in combination with ritonavir 200 mg bid. Take with food	Drug-drug interaction profile more complex than other PI's; check package insert carefully. Use with caution in patients with known sulfa allergy. Avoid in patients with coagulopathies

Table 3.1. Antiretroviral Agents Used for HIV Infection (cont'd)

Drug (abbreviation; trade name, manufacturer)	Formulations	Usual Adult Dosing§	Comments
Darunavir (DRV; Prezista, Tibotec Therapeutics)	300-, 600-mg tablets; 400-mg (approval pending)	600 mg bid with ritonavir 100 mg bid (treatment experienced); 800 mg qd with ritonavir 100 mg qd (treatment naive)	Use with caution in patients with known sulfa allergy
		FUSION INHIBITOR	
Enfuvirtide (T-20; Fuzeon, Roche)‡	Injectable (lyophilized powder). Each single-use vial contains 108 mg of enfuvirtide to be reconstituted with 1.1 mL of sterile water for injection for delivery of approximately 90 mg/mL	90 mg bid IV. Administered subcutaneously into upper arm, anterior thigh, or abdomen	Each injection should be administered at a site different from the preceding injection site and only where there is no current injection site reaction from an earlier dose. Should not be injected into moles, scar tissue, bruises, or the navel
		CCR5 ANTAGONIST	
Maraviroc (MVC; Selzentry, Pfizer)	150-, 300-mg tablets	150 mg, 300 mg or 600 bid depending on concomitant drugs (see p. 170 for details); may be taken with or without food	Testing for viral tropism recommended before use – only active against R5-tropic virus. Dose-related hypotension may occur. Monitor for hepatotoxicity
		INTEGRASE INHIBITOR	
Raltegravir (RAL; Isentress, Merck)	400-mg tablet	One 400-mg tablet bid with or without food	Rifampin decreases plasma concentrations of raltegravir – use with caution

* Nevirapine and efavirenz are cytochrome p450 cyp3A4 inducers; delavirdine is an inhibitor. Consult package insert for full drug interaction profile

† All protease inhibitors are hepatically metabolized by the cytochrome p450 system; they also are specific inhibitors of cyp3A4 and have induction effects on other enzymes. Consult package insert for full drug-drug interaction profile

‡ Consult package insert for full drug interaction profile

§ See Chapter 9 for dosing adjustments in renal or hepatic insufficiency. Unless otherwise stated, medication may be taken with or without food

SELECTION OF AN OPTIMAL INITIAL ANTIRETROVIRAL REGIMEN (Tables 3.2-3.5)

Selection of the optimal initial antiretroviral regimen must take into consideration antiviral potency, tolerability, and safety. In the DHHS and IAS-USA Guidelines (Tables 3.3, 3.4), all recommended regimens consist of three active agents: an NRTI pair (containing 3TC or FTC as one of the drugs) plus either an NNRTI or a PI. As such, choosing a specific regimen therefore can be reduced to four major decisions (see Table 3.2).

Table 3.2. Major Decisions in Selecting the Initial Antiretroviral Regimen*

Decision	Comment
What is the optimal NRTI to pair with 3TC or FTC	Because of the availability of once-daily, fixed-dose formulations and a low risk of lipoatrophy, many clinicians are currently choosing either TDF (co-formulated with FTC as Truvada) or ABC (co-formulated with 3TC as Epzicom). ABC therapy should be preceded by testing for HLA-B*5701 to reduce the risk of ABC hypersensitivity.
Should the third drug be an NNRTI or a PI	NNRTI-based regimens – in particular those containing EFV – are in general simpler to take than PI-based treatments. EFV-based regimens have also demonstrated superior antiviral activity in most prospective clinical trials (Riddler SA , et al. XVI International AIDS Conference 2006; Abstract THLB0204.). However, PI-based therapy is required in patients with baseline NNRTI resistance. While PI-based regimens have a somewhat higher pill burden, they confer a lower risk of resistance in the case of virologic failure.
If an NNRTI-based regimen is chosen, which agent should be used	In general, EFV is the preferred NNRTI due to comparable or superior antiviral activity to all comparators in prospective clinical trials. It is also available as a single-tablet triple regimen combined with TDF and FTC. However, EFV should be avoided in women of childbearing potential who may wish to become pregnant and may be difficult to tolerate for patients with psychiatric disease. In these contexts, NVP would be preferred, so long as the baseline CD4 cell count does not exceed $250/mm^3$ in a woman or $400/mm^3$ in a man.
If a PI-based regimen is chosen, which PI should be used	There are more options for PI-based than for NNRTI-based therapy. In general, RTV-boosted PI's provide the best combination of simplicity and antiviral potency. These include LPV/r (given once or twice daily), ATV/r, FPV/r, or SQV/r. DRV/r will also be an option at a dose of 800/100 mg daily once the 400-mg tablet of DRV is approved.

* All recommended regimens consist of three active agents: an NRTI pair (containing 3TC or FTC as one of the drugs) plus either an NNRTI or a PI. Information on adverse drug reactions and drug-drug interactions highlight important differences between available agents. Combinations not listed as "Preferred" or "Alternative" regimens in Tables 3.3 and 3.4 should in general be avoided.

Table 3.3. Antiretroviral Components Recommended for Treatment of HIV-1 Infection in Treatment Naive Patients: DHHS Guidelines*

SELECT NRTI PAIR PLUS EITHER NNRTI OR PI			
	NRTI Pair	**NNRTI**	**PI**
Preferred	• Abacavir/lamivudine[†,¶] (if negative for HLAB*5701) • Tenofovir/emtricitabine[†,¶]	• Efavirenz[‡]	• Atazanavir + ritonavir • Fosamprenavir + ritonavir (2x/d) • Lopinavir/ritonavir[¶] (2x/d)
Alternative	• Zidovudine/lamivudine[†,¶] • Didanosine + (emtricitabine or lamivudine)	• Nevirapine[#]	• Atazanavir** • Fosamprenavir • Fosamprenavir + ritonavir (1x/d) • Lopinavir/ritonavir[¶] (1x/d) • Saquinavir + ritonavir

* A combination antiretroviral regimen in treatment-naive patients generally contains 1 NNRTI + 2 NRTI's, or a single or ritonavir-boosted PI + 2 NRTI's. Selection of a regimen for an antiretroviral-naive patient should be individualized based on virologic efficacy, toxicities, pill burden, dosing frequency, drug-drug interaction potential, and co-morbid conditions. Components listed above are designated as preferred when clinical trial data suggest optimal and durable efficacy with acceptable tolerability and ease of use. Alternative components are those that clinical trial data show efficacy but that have disadvantages, such as antiviral activity or toxicities, compared with the preferred agent. In some cases, for an individual patient, a component listed as alternative may actually be the preferred component. Options listed in the table appear in alphabetical order, except for "Alternative, NRTI Pair," which appear in order of preference. For antiretroviral regimens in the HIV-infected pregnant patient, see http://aidsinfo.nih.gov/guidelines.

† Emtricitabine may be used in place of lamivudine and vice versa.

‡ Efavirenz is not recommended for use in the first trimester of pregnancy or in sexually active women with child-bearing potential who are not using effective contraception.

¶ Co-formulated.

Nevirapine should not be initiated in women with CD4 > 250 cells/mm^3 or in men with CD4 > 400 cells/mm^3 because of increased risk of symptomatic hepatic events.

** Atazanavir must be boosted with ritonavir if used in combination with tenofovir.

Adapted from: Panel on Clinical Practices for Treatment of HIV Infection. Guidelines for the use of Antiretroviral Agents in HIV-Infected Adults and Adolescents. Department of Health and Human Services. January 29, 2008. www.hivatis.org

Table 3.4. Initial Antiretroviral Regimens: International AIDS Society - USA Treatment Guidelines

SELECT NRTI PAIR PLUS EITHER NNRTI OR PI			
	NRTI Pair‡	NNRTI	PI
Recommended	• Tenofovir/emtricitabine§,¶ • Zidovudine/lamivudine§,¶ • Abacavir/lamivudine§,¶	• Efavirenz* • Nevirapine†	• Lopinavir/ritonavir¶ • Atazanavir + ritonavir • Saquinavir + ritonavir • Fosamprenavir + ritonavir

* See footnote ‡, Table 3.3 (p. 28).
† See footnote #, Table 3.3 (p. 27).
‡ Triple-NRTI regimens are no longer recommended as initial therapy because of insufficient antiretroviral potency compared with a regimen containing efavirenz. However, for patients requiring treatment with regimens that preclude use of NNRTI's or PI's, a combination consisting of zidovudine, abacavir, and lamivudine may be considered
§ Emtricitabine may be used in place of lamivudine and vice versa.
¶ Co-formulated.
Adapted from: JAMA 2006;296:827-843

Table 3.5. Selected Antiretroviral Therapy Options

ART/Combination	Advantages	Disadvantages
	NRTI COMBINATIONS	
Emtricitabine 200 mg (PO) qd + tenofovir 300 mg (PO) qd	Compared favorably to d4T/3TC (tolerability) and ZDV/3TC (tolerability and efficacy) in prospective clinical trials (JAMA 2004;292:191-201, N Engl J Med 2006;354:251-60). Low risk of lipoatrophy. Available as part of triple-combination therapy with efavirenz (Atripla)	Lowers atazanavir levels; must use RTV boosting. May cause renal dysfunction (rare)
Lamivudine 300 mg (PO) qd + abacavir 300 mg (PO) bid (or 600 mg [PO] qd)	Combination tablet (Epzicom). Once-daily dosing (1 pill per day). Better CD4 response than ZDV/3TC. Low risk of lipoatrophy	Abacavir hypersensitivity; need for pretreatment screening test (HLA-B*5701) to reduce risk. Hepatic dysfunction is a relative contradiction. Abacavir treatment may be associated with an increased risk of MI (Lancet 2008, April 1, e-pub)
Zidovudine 300 mg (PO) bid + lamivudine 150 mg (PO) bid	Fixed-dose combination tablet (Combivir) reduces pill burden. ZDV especially effective in treating ITP and has relatively good CNS penetration	ZDV has highest rate of subjective side effects (nausea, GI disturbance, headache) in NRTI class and is the most marrow suppressive. Long-term use associated with lipoatrophy
Stavudine 40 mg (PO) bid + lamivudine 150 mg (PO) bid or emtricitabine 200 mg (PO) qd	Excellent initial tolerability	d4T-based regimens associated with higher rates of hyperlipidemia, neuropathy, lipodystrophy

Table 3.5. Selected Antiretroviral Therapy Options (cont'd)

ART/Combination	Advantages	Disadvantages
	NRTI COMBINATIONS (cont'd)	
Lamivudine 300 mg (PO) qd (or emtricitabine 200 mg [PO] qd) + didanosine 400 mg (PO) qd	Once-daily dosing	Limited long-term data. ddI must be taken on an empty stomach
Zidovudine 300 mg (PO) bid + lamivudine 150 mg (PO) bid + abacavir 300 mg (PO) bid	Defers protease inhibitor and NNRTI regimens. Fixed-dose combination tablet (Trizivir) has low pill burden (1 pill bid). On its own, few drug-drug interactions	Abacavir hypersensitivity in 3-8%. As triple therapy, significantly lower virologic efficacy compared with efavirenz-based regimens
	PROTEASE INHIBITORS	
Atazanavir 400 mg (PO) qd, or 300 mg qd + ritonavir 100 mg qd. (Ritonavir-boosting required with efavirenz, tenofovir, or in PI-experienced patients)	Only once daily protease inhibitor, low pill burden; low rate of GI side effects; neutral or minimal effect on plasma lipids. Early virologic failure associated with 150L mutation – other PI's remain active. Non-inferior to LPV/r when combined with TDF/FTC (15th CROI 2008, abstract #37)	Mild indirect hyperbilirubinemia frequent; when given unboosted (without ritonavir), less active than lopinavir/ritonavir in protease-inhibitor experienced patients; first-degree AV block may occur (not advanced heart block); absorption reduced when given with acid reducing therapy
Darunavir 600 mg (PO) bid with ritonavir 100 mg (PO) bid (treatment-experienced); darunavir 800 mg (PO) qd with ritonavir 100 mg (PO) qd (treatment-naive)	More active than comparator PIs in treatment-experienced patients (Lancet 2007;369:1169-78, Lancet 2007;370:49-58). Non-inferior to LPV/r in treatment-naive patients, with greater efficacy than LPV/r once-daily (Dejesus E, 47th Interscience Conference on Antimicrobial Agents and Chemotherapy, 2007, Abstract H-718b.)	Contains sulfonamide moiety; use with caution in patients with sulfa allergy
Fosamprenavir: *PI naive*: 1400 mg bid (or 1400 mg qd with ritonavir 200 mg qd). *PI experienced*: 700 mg bid with ritonavir 100 mg bid	More active than nelfinavir in head-to head studies (AIDS 2004;18:1529-37, J AIDS 2004;35:22-32); relatively low rates of GI side effects. Non-inferior to LPV/r soft-gel capsules in treatment-naive patients in prospective study (Lancet 2006;368:476-82)	Rash may occur somewhat more commonly than with other PI's. Contains sulfonamide moiety; use with caution in patients with sulfa allergy. When given bid with ritonavir, GI side effects and lipids comparable to LPV/r
Indinavir 800 mg (PO) q8h	Good CNS penetration	Q8h dosing on empty stomach is required. Nephrolithiasis, paronychia, dry skin are distinctive side effects to this agent. Can be given with low-dose ritonavir for twice-daily dosing (indinavir 800 mg bid plus ritonavir 100 mg bid), but optimal dose is not clear and adverse effects are often increased

Table 3.5. Selected Antiretroviral Therapy Options (cont'd)

ART/Combination	Advantages	Disadvantages
	PROTEASE INHIBITORS (cont'd)	
Lopinavir + ritonavir (Kaletra) tablet formulation (lopinavir 200 mg/ritonavir 50 mg) dosed as 2 tablets bid or 4 tablets qd	More effective than nelfinavir when combined with d4T and 3TC in randomized, double-blind trial (Walmsley, N Engl J Med;346:2039, 2002). Generally well tolerated. Virologic rebound usually associated with no PI resistance. Only PI co-formulated with ritonavir	Associated with hyperlipidemia (especially hypertriglyceridemia). Diarrhea and nausea are the most common adverse effects
Nelfinavir 1250 mg (PO) bid	Early virologic failure often associated with unique D30N mutation, allowing "salvage" with other protease inhibitors	Diarrhea may be severe for some patients. Less potent than boosted PI's. Markedly decreased absorption if taken without food
Saquinavir 1000 mg (PO) bid + ritonavir 100 mg bid	Pill burden reduced (3 pills twice daily including ritonavir) by new saquinavir 500 mg hard-gel formulation (Invirase)	Limited long-term data in comparative clinical trials. Higher pill burden than other preferred PI options
Tipranavir 500 mg (PO) bid + ritonavir 200 (PO) mg bid	PI with activity against highly PI-resistant strains, with greater viral load reduction than non-darunavir comparator boosted PI's	Higher rates of hepatitis and hyperlipidemia than comparator boosted PI's. Complex drug interaction profile. Cannot be co-administered with other PI's due to reduced plasma levels. Reports of intracerebral hemorrhage; avoid in patients with coagulopathies
	NNRTI's	
Delavirdine 400 mg (PO) q8h	Can be taken with or without food. Inhibits p450 enzymes and can act as a pharmaco-kinetic booster for some protease inhibitors, most notably indinavir	Highest pill burden and most frequent dosing in drug class. Rash in 18%, though usually mild. Single mutation leads to high-level resistance. Rarely used
Efavirenz 600 mg (PO) qd	Long half-life (60 hours) allows once-daily dosing. Superior to comparators in multiple clinical trials (N Engl J Med 1999;341:1865-73; N Engl J Med 2004;350:1850-61; Lancet 2004;363:1253-63). Proven efficacy in patients with high HIV RNA and advanced disease (J Infect Dis 2008;197:1006-10); available as part of single pill triple ART (Atripla)	Near-universal CNS disturbances (vivid dreams, daytime somnolence, dizziness) at outset of therapy (usually abates with time). Rash in ~ 20% (can generally can treat through). Not to be used in pregnancy (pregnancy category D). Single mutation leads to high-level resistance

Table 3.5. Selected Antiretroviral Therapy Options (cont'd)

ART/Combination	Advantages	Disadvantages
	NNRTI's (cont'd)	
Nevirapine 200 mg (PO) qd x 14 days, then 200 mg (PO) bid	Low pill-burden. Can be taken with or without food	Relatively high rate of hepatotoxicity and severe dermatologic/systemic reactions, more common in women with CD4 > 250 and men with CD4 > 400; may be used with caution in pregnancy. Rate of Stevens-Johnson syndrome ~ 1%. Single mutation leads to high-level resistance
Etravirine 200 mg (PO) bid	Retains activity against most NNRTI-resistant viruses, including those harboring the K103N mutation. Highly effective when coadministered with DRV/r in treatment-experienced patients (Lancet 2007;370:29-48)	High pill burden for this drug class; FDA-approved for twice-daily dosing only (PK would support once-daily). Exposure decreased 50% when taken without food. Rash in 15-20%. Cannot be given with some PI's, notably ATV/r, TPV/r, or any PI without ritonavir boosting
	FUSION INHIBITOR	
Enfuvirtide 90 mg (SQ) bid	Produces further ↓ in HIV RNA and ↑ in CD4 in multiple-treatment experienced patients when given with an optimized background regimen (J AIDS 2005;40:413-21). No cross resistance with other antiretrovirals.	Requires twice-daily subcutaneous injection; induces injection site reactions of varying severity; more expensive than other antiretroviral agents
	CCR5 ANTAGONIST	
Maraviroc 150 mg or 300 mg or 600 mg (PO) bid	Novel mechanism of action, hence no cross-resistance with other drug classes. When combined with an optimized background regimen, more active than placebo in highly treatment experienced patients (14th Conference on Retroviruses and Opp Infections 2007, Abstract 104aLB). May stimulate better CD4 responses than comparator drugs	Multiple dosing recommendations depending on coadministered antiretrovirals. Less effective than EFV in treatment-naive patients (Saag M, et al. 4th, IAS Conference on HIV Pathogenesis, Treatment and Prevention, 2007, Abstract # WESS104). Requires pretreatment assessment of viral tropism, a costly test with relatively slow turnaround time (~ 3 weeks). Approximately 50% of treatment-experienced patients will not be candidates due to presence of dual-mixed or X4 tropic virus. Patients incorrectly classified as having R5 tropic virus who are treated with maraviroc will have selection of X4 virus, which may be more pathogenic. Concerns about hepatotoxicity and possible oncogenicity based on results of studies with other drugs in CCR5 inhibitor class. Cellular target - may be immunomodulatory

Table 3.5. Selected Antiretroviral Therapy Options (cont'd)

ART/Combination	Advantages	Disadvantages
	INTEGRASE INHIBITOR	
Raltegravir 400 mg (PO) bid	Novel mechanism of action, hence no cross-resistance with existing drug classes. When combined with an optimized background regimen, more active than placebo in highly treatment experienced patients (Cooper D, et al, CROI 2008, Boston, MA, abstract 788). Compared with EFV in treatment-naive patients when combined with TDF and 3TC, raltegravir was just as effective and induced a faster HIV RNA decline (Markowitz M, J Acquir Immune Defic Syndr 2007;46:125-33). Few drug-drug interactions	Twice-daily dosing. Virologic failure associated with relatively rapid development of integrase inhibitor resistance. Levels significantly lowered by rifampin – clinical relevance unclear

HIV THERAPY AND LIPODYSTROPHY SYNDROME

The metabolic and morphologic changes that occur with HIV therapy are sometimes grouped under the term "lipodystrophy syndrome." Key features include *subcutaneous lipoatrophy,* which is most evident in the face, limbs, and buttocks; and *regional fat accumulation*, which may occur in the posterior or anterior portions of the neck, as well as the in midsection, as a manifestation of visceral adiposity. Patients may have predominantly lipoatrophy – the most common abnormality – fat accumulation, or both. These morphologic changes are often accompanied by metabolic derangements, including lipid dysregulation (increased triglycerides and total cholesterol; reduced HDL cholesterol) and insulin resistance. The etiology of the lipodystrophy syndrome is poorly understood, and there are clearly both host and treatment factors.

A. Lipoatrophy

1. **Overview.** Lipoatrophy is the most common morphologic abnormality in HIV disease. The most important host risk factors is the stage of HIV disease, as patients with more advanced HIV-related immunosuppression are at greatest risk. Among treatment-related factors, the leading hypothesis is that NRTI-induced mitochondrial toxicity induces fat cell apoptosis, and NRTI's with the highest *in vitro* inhibition of the mitochondrial enzyme polymerase gamma pose the greatest risk. Based on this hypothesis, a hierarchy of treatment-associated risk for lipoatrophy would be as follows: *highest risk* for dideoxynucleosides (stavudine, didanosine, and zalcitabine); *intermediate risk* for zidovudine; and *lowest risk* for tenofovir, abacavir, lamivudine, and emtricitabine. While one study showed a

greater degree of mild lipoatrophy with efavirenz versus lopinavir/r treatment, in general the NNRTI class of medications has not been implicated in this process.

2. **Treatment.** Treatment strategies for lipoatrophy consist of drug substitutions, insulin sensitizing agents, and plastic surgery. Substituting tenofovir or abacavir for stavudine or zidovudine leads to a gradual increase in limb fat that is often accompanied by a subjective improvement in facial appearance (AIDS 2006;20:2043-50). Such improvements occur slowly after antiretroviral switches and may not be evident to the patient for several months. The tenofovir substitution strategy may also improve lipid abnormalities. Substituting an NNRTI for the PI-component of the regimen has had no consistent effect on morphologic changes (AIDS 2005;19:917-25). Although there was initial optimism that insulin sensitizing agents – in particular rosiglitazone – would help reverse lipoatrophy, the bulk of prospective data do not support a role for this approach, and it is not recommended in the absence of insulin resistance. Finally, plastic surgery for facial lipoatrophy can often dramatically improve appearance. The most common approach is injection of biologically inert substances such as polylactic acid (Sculptra). Patient satisfaction after polylactic acid injections is extremely high, and thus far the procedure appears safe. The major drawbacks to this treatment approach include the lack of long-term efficacy and safety data, relatively high cost, and lack of effect on lipoatrophy of the arms and legs. Patients should be informed that most insurance policies and state-funded programs will not cover the cost of polylactic acid injections.

B. Fat Accumulation

1. **Overview.** Fat accumulation occurs less commonly than fat atrophy, but can be highly disfiguring. The neck, upper body, and intra-abdominal (visceral) sites are most often involved. (Neck fat accumulation in the posterior compartment is often referred to as a buffalo hump.) Despite the similarity to Cushing's Syndrome, serum cortisol levels are not elevated. While fat accumulation syndrome is most strongly linked to PI-based therapy, cases have occurred in the absence of PI's as well.
2. **Treatment.** No treatment modification has consistently led to improvement. Exercise may reduce central fat accumulation, and weight loss may reduce neck fat, but improvements are generally modest. Liposuction of neck fat accumulation is the most rapidly effective technique, but recurrences may occur. Insurance coverage for neck liposuction can sometimes be arranged if the fat accumulation leads to medical problems such as neck pain or sleep apnea.

C. Prevention of Lipodystrophy. Since morphologic changes are only slowly reversible and may be permanent in some patients, the best strategy is to choose treatments that are least likely to induce these abnormalities. Of currently preferred NRTI combinations, tenofovir/emtricitabine and abacavir/lamivudine induce less fat atrophy than zidovudine/lamivudine (Table 3.6). In addition, providers should consider a

Table 3.6. Treatment and Prevention of Body Habitus Changes Associated with Antiretroviral Therapy

Treatment	• Substitute tenofovir or abacavir for thymidine analogue • Polylactic acid injections for facial lipoatrophy • Weight loss and exercise for fat accumulation • Liposuction for dorsocervical fat accumulation
Prevention	• Start therapy before advanced HIV disease • Select initial NRTI backbones less likely to induce lipoatrophy (i.e., emtricitabine/tenofovir or abacavir/lamivudine) • Consider pro-active switch to tenofovir DF or abacavir for patients still on thymidine analogues (ZDV or d4T)

proactive switching strategy for patients receiving long-term zidovudine/lamivudine. Regimens containing stavudine should be avoided unless there are no alternatives. The morphologic changes associated with didanosine + lamivudine are not well defined but, as noted above, didanosine has a relatively high degree of mitochondrial toxicity *in vitro*, and this correlates with increased risk of fat atrophy.

D. Lipid Abnormalities. Multiple abnormalities in lipid metabolism were reported in HIV-infected patients before the availability of PI-based antiretroviral therapy, including increased levels of very low-density lipoprotein (VLDL) cholesterol and triglycerides and decreased levels of high-density lipoprotein (HDL) cholesterol, low-density lipoprotein (LDL) cholesterol, and apolipoprotein B (JAMA 2003;289:2978-82). However, soon after the introduction of PI's, a dramatic increase in triglyceride levels and, to a lesser extent, total cholesterol levels were evident in PI-treated patients.

1. **Antiretroviral Therapy and Dyslipidemia.** The PI's ritonavir, indinavir, saquinavir, nelfinavir, lopinavir/r, and tipranavir are all associated to varying degrees with clinically-significant dyslipidemia. Saquinavir, unboosted fosamprenavir, and in particular atazanavir are more lipid neutral; however, ritonavir boosting worsens lipid profile even of these PI's. Other components of the antiretroviral regimen may also induce lipid disturbances: d4T and ZDV are both more likely to raise lipids than tenofovir, and efavirenz increases lipids, especially triglycerides, more than nevirapine. Treatment of HIV may have the favorable effect of raising HDL cholesterol, particularly with nevirapine and efavirenz.
2. **Treatment of Dyslipidemia.** Various approaches can be taken to treat PI-associated dyslipidemia. As for HIV-negative patients, the first step consists of therapeutic lifestyle changes, including dietary counseling, reduction in alcohol intake, smoking cessation, and increased aerobic exercise. Unfortunately, lifestyle changes alone are often insufficient to reverse lipid abnormalities in patients with HIV. The two most widely used pharmacological strategies are substitution of the potentially offending antiretroviral agent with an alternative antiretroviral, or use

of lipid-modifying drug therapy. In patients who are virologicaly suppressed and have no or little presumed antiretroviral resistance, the former strategy is generally safe but may not lower lipids into the desirable range (AIDS 2005;19:1051-8). When switching antiretroviral drugs it is important to weigh the risks of new treatment-related toxicities and virologic relapse against the risks of potential drug interactions and new treatment-related toxicities from lipid-lowering agents. Table 3.7 cites some potential switch strategies; if there is more than one possible offending agent, the changes should be made sequentially to ensure that the initial change is well-tolerated. The use of lipid-lowering agents in HIV-infected patients is notable for a relative lack of efficacy and a high risk of drug interactions, particularly between the statins and PI's. Nonetheless, lipid abnormalities should be aggressively treated just as in HIV-negative patients, especially when other cardiac risk factors are present.

Elevations in LDL cholesterol will usually require statin therapy. Most of the statins, with the exception of pravastatin, fluvastatin and rosuvastatin, are metabolized by the cytochrome P450 enzyme system via the 3A4 isoform (CYP3A4). Most PI's inhibit CYP3A4, potentially leading to elevated statin levels and increased the risk of statin-related toxicity, including rhabdomyolysis (Clin Infect Dis 2002;35:e111-2). Due to absence of PI-drug interactions, pravastatin is the statin of choice when treating PI-related dyslipidemia. If lipid targets are not met with pravastatin, atorvastatin — a more potent agent — is an acceptable alternative, so long as the starting dose is 10 mg daily and the patient is closely monitored for hepatic/muscle toxicity. Fluvastatin and rosuvastatin, which are also not metabolized via CYP3A4, may be other acceptable options, although studies evaluating their use in HIV patients are more limited than with pravastatin or atorvastatin. When hypertriglyceridemia is the predominant abnormality, a fibrate such as gemfibrozil or fenofibrate should be tried first. As for HIV-negative patients, refractory elevations in triglycerides may respond to fish oil preparations.

Table 3.7. Drug-Induced Dyslipidemia and Switch Therapy

Cause	Switch To	Comments
Protease inhibitors (PI's): ritonavir, indinavir, saquinavir, nelfinavir, lopinavir/r, tipranavir	Atazanavir or atazanavir/ritonavir	Need to use boosted atazanavir if patient is also on tenofovir. If patient is on a proton pump inhibitor, atazanavir should in general be avoided
d4T or ZDV	Tenofovir	Use with caution in patients with impaired renal function; reduce dose per package insert guidelines
Efavirenz	Nevirapine	Avoid in women with CD4 > 250/mm^3 or men with CD4 > 400/mm^3 due to increased risk of hepatotoxicity

ANTIRETROVIRAL THERAPY AND POTENTIALLY LIFE-THREATENING ADVERSE EFFECTS

This section was adapted from Guidelines for the Use of Antiretroviral Agents in HIV-Infected Adults and Adolescents, Department of Health and Human Services, www.aidsinfo.nih.gov/guidelines, January 29, 2008.

Acute Hepatic Failure

A. Causative Agent. Nevirapine

B. Clinical Presentation. Onset: Greatest risk within first few weeks of therapy; can occur through 18 weeks. Symptoms: Abrupt onset of flu-like symptoms (nausea, vomiting, myalgia, fatigue), abdominal pain, jaundice, or fever with or without skin rash; may progress to fulminant hepatic failure with encephalopathy. Approximately 50% of cases have accompanying skin rash. Some may present as part of DRESS syndrome (drug rash with eosinophilia and systemic symptoms).

C. Frequency. 4% overall (2.5-11% from different trials). In women: 11% in those with pre-NVP CD4 > 250/mm^3 vs. 0.9% with CD4 < 250/mm^3. In men: 6.3% with pre-NVP CD4 > 400/mm^3 vs. 2.3% with CD4 < 400/mm^3.

D. Risk Factors. Higher CD4 cell count at initiation (> 250/mm^3 in women; > 400/mm^3 in men); female gender (including pregnant women); elevated ALT or AST at baseline; HBV or HCV co-infection; alcoholic liver disease; HIV-negative individuals when NVP is used for post-exposure prophylaxis; high NVP concentration. Treatment-experienced patients with high CD4 cell counts appear to be at lower risk than those who are treatment naive.

E. Prevention/Monitoring. Avoid initiation of NVP in women with CD4 > 250/mm^3 or men with CD4 > 400/mm^3 unless the benefit clearly outweighs the risk. Counsel patients regarding signs and symptoms of hepatitis, and instruct patients to stop NVP and seek medical attention for signs and symptoms of hepatitis, severe skin rash, or hypersensitivity reactions. Monitor ALT/AST every 2 weeks during first month of NVP, then monthly x 3 months, then every 3 months. Obtain ALT/AST in patients with rash. Two-week dose escalation may reduce incidence of hepatic events.

F. Management. Discontinue antiretrovirals including nevirapine (caution should be taken in discontinuation of 3TC, FTC, or TDF in HBV co-infected patients). Discontinue all other hepatotoxic agents if possible. Rule out other causes of hepatitis. Provide aggressive supportive care as indicated. Note: Hepatic injury may progress despite treatment discontinuation. Careful monitoring should continue until symptom resolution. **Do not rechallenge patient with NVP**. The safety of other NNRTI's (EFV, ETV, or DLV) in patients who experienced significant hepatic event from NVP is unknown–use with caution.

Lactic Acidosis/Hepatic Steatosis ± Pancreatitis (severe mitochondrial toxicities)

A. Causative Agents. NRTI's, especially d4T, ddI, ZDV

B. Clinical Presentation. Onset: Months after initiation of NRTI's. Symptoms: Initial onset may be insidious with nonspecific GI prodrome (nausea, anorexia, abdominal pain, vomiting), weight loss, fatigue. Subsequent symptoms may be rapidly progressive with tachycardia, tachypnea, hyperventilation, jaundice, muscular weakness, mental status changes, or respiratory distress. Some may present with multi-organ failure, such as fulminant hepatic failure, acute pancreatitis, encephalopathy, respiratory failure. Laboratory findings: Increased lactate (often > 5 mmol); low arterial pH (some < 7.0); low serum bicarbonate; increased anion gap; elevated serum transaminases, prothrombin time, and bilirubin; low serum albumin. Increased serum amylase and lipase in patients with pancreatitis. Histologic findings of the liver show microvesicular or macrovesicular steatosis.

C. Frequency. Rare. One estimate 0.85 cases per 1000 patient-years. Mortality up to 50% in some case series (especially in patients with serum lactate > 10 mmol)

D. Risk Factors. d4T + ddI; d4T, ZDV, ddI (d4T most frequently implicated); long duration of NRTI use; female gender; obesity; pregnancy (especially d4T + ddI); ddI + hydroxyurea or ribavirin; high baseline body mass index.

E. Prevention/Monitoring. Routine monitoring of lactic acid is not recommended. Consider obtaining lactate levels in patients with low serum bicarbonate or a high anion gap and complaints consistent with lactic acidosis. (Employ appropriate phlebotomy technique for obtaining lactate level, avoid prolonged use of tourniquet, process promptly.)

F. Management. Discontinue all antiretrovirals if syndrome is highly suspected (diagnosis established by clinical correlation, drug history, and lactate level). Administer symptomatic support with fluid hydration. Some patients may require IV bicarbonate infusion, hemodialysis or hemofiltration, parenteral nutrition or mechanical ventilation. IV thiamine and/or riboflavin have resulted in rapid resolution of hyperlactatemia in some case reports. Note: Interpretation of high lactate level should be done in the context of clinical findings. The implication of asymptomatic hyperlactatemia is unknown at this point, and one study found this entity to be rare if specimens are collected properly. Consider using NRTI's with less mitochondrial toxicity (e.g., ABC, TDF, 3TC, FTC) *after* lactate levels return to normal (closely monitor serum bicarbonate and lactate after restarting NRTI's). Some consider using NRTI–sparing regimens with PI + NNRTI ± fusion inhibitor (e.g., IDV + EFV, LPV/r + EFV); efficacy and benefit of this type of regimen is unknown but currently under investigation.

Lactic Acidosis/Rapidly Progressive Ascending Neuromuscular Weakness

A. Causative Agent. d4T most frequently implicated.

B. Clinical Presentation. Onset: Months after initiation of ART, then dramatic motor weakness occurring within days to weeks. Symptoms: Very rapidly progressive ascending demyelinating polyneuropathy (can mimic Guillain-Barre Syndrome). Some develop respiratory paralysis requiring mechanical ventilation. Can be fatal. Laboratory findings: Low arterial pH, increased lactate, low serum bicarbonate, increased anion gap, markedly increased creatine phosphokinase.

C. Frequency. Rare.

D. Risk Factors. Prolonged d4T use (found in 61 of 69 [88%] cases in one report).

E. Prevention/Monitoring. Early recognition and discontinuation of antiretrovirals may avoid further progression.

F. Management. Discontinue antiretroviral therapy and provide supportive care, including mechanical ventilation if needed. Other measures attempted with variable successes include plasmapheresis, high-dose corticosteroids, intravenous immunoglobulin, carnitine, acetylcarnitine. Recovery often takes months, ranging from complete recovery to substantial residual deficits. Symptoms may be irreversible in some patients. **Do not rechallenge patient with offending agent.**

Stevens-Johnson Syndrome/Toxic Epidermal Necrosis

A. Causative Agents. NVP > EFV, DLV, ETV. Also reported with APV, f-APV, ABC, ZDV, ddI, IDV, LPV/r, ATV.

B. Clinical Presentation. Onset: First few days to weeks after initiation of therapy. Symptoms: Skin eruption with mucosal ulcerations (may involve orogingival mucosa, conjunctiva, anogenital area); can rapidly evolve with blister or bullae formation, and may eventually evolve to epidermal detachment and/or necrosis. For NVP, may occur with hepatic toxicity. Systemic symptoms include fever, tachycardia, malaise, myalgia, arthralgia. Complications include dehydration, bacterial or fungal superinfection, multiorgan system failure.

C. Frequency. NVP 0.3-1%; DLV and EFV 0.1%; ETV < 0.1%. 1-2 case reports for ABC, f-APV, ddI, ZDV, IDV, LPV/r, ATV.

D. Risk Factors. For NVP: female, Black, Asian, Hispanic.

E. Prevention/Monitoring. Titrate NVP: always start with 200 mg once daily x 2 weeks, then escalate to 200 mg bid. Instruct patients to report symptoms as soon as they appear. Avoid use of corticosteroids during NVP dose escalation (may increase incidence of rash).

F. Management. Discontinue all antiretrovirals and any other possible offending agents (e.g., cotrimoxazole). Aggressive symptomatic support may include intensive care support, aggressive local wound care (e.g., in a burn unit), intravenous hydration, parenteral nutrition, pain management, antipyretics, and empiric broad-spectrum antimicrobial therapy if superinfection is suspected. Controversial management strategies include corticosteroids, IV immunoglobulin. **Do not rechallenge patient with offending agent.** It is unknown whether patients who experienced SJS while taking an NNRTI are more susceptible to SJS when another NNRTI is used; most experts would avoid use of this class unless no other option is available.

Hypersensitivity Reaction

A. Causative Agent. ABC.

B. Clinical Presentation. Onset of initial reaction: Median onset 9 days; 90% within first 6 weeks. Onset of rechallenge reactions: Within hours of rechallenge dose. Symptoms: Acute onset of symptoms (in descending frequency): high fever, diffuse skin rash, malaise, nausea, headache, myalgia, chills, diarrhea, vomiting, abdominal pain, dyspnea, arthralgia, respiratory symptoms (pharyngitis, dyspnea/tachypnea). With continuation of ABC, symptoms may worsen to include hypotension, respiratory distress, vascular collapse. Rechallenge reactions are generally of greater intensity than the initial reaction and can mimic anaphylaxis.

C. **Frequency.** Approximately 8% in clinical trial (2-9%); 5% in retrospective analysis; significantly reduced with pretreatment HLA screening. Less common in patients of African descent.

D. **Risk Factors.** Prospective and retrospective clinical studies have demonstrated a strong link between the presence HLA-B*5701 and the occurrence of ABC hypersensitivity reaction (Mallal S, N Engl J Med 2008;358:568-79). Approximately 50% of HLA-B*5701 positive patients will develop an ABC hypersensitivity reaction, and hence the drug should not be used in these individuals. In patients negative for this haplotype, immunologically-confirmed ABC hypersensitivity reactions have not yet been reported (although other allergic reactions still may occur).

E. **Prevention/Monitoring.** Before use of abacavir, all patients should undergo testing for HLA-B*5701, and patients testing positive for HLA-B*5701 should be labelled as allergic to abacavir in their medical records. Educate patients about potential signs and symptoms of hypersensitivity reactions and the need to immediately report symptoms. A wallet card with warning information is useful for patients.

F. **Management.** Discontinue ABC and other antiretrovirals. Rule out other causes of symptoms (e.g., intercurrent illnesses such as viral syndromes, and other causes of skin rash). Most signs and symptoms resolve 48 hours after discontinuation of ABC. For more severe cases provide symptomatic support with antipyretics, fluid resuscitation, pressure support (if necessary). **Do not rechallenge patients with ABC after suspected hypersensitivity reaction.**

ANTIRETROVIRAL THERAPY AND OTHER POTENTIALLY SERIOUS ADVERSE EFFECTS

This section was adapted from Guidelines for the Use of Antiretroviral Agents in HIV-Infected Adults and Adolescents, Department of Health and Human Services, www.aidsinfo.nih.gov/guidelines, October 10, 2006.

Bleeding Episodes

A. **Causative Agents.** TPV/r: reports of intracranial hemorrhage (ICH). PI's: increased bleeding in hemophiliac patients.

B. **Clinical Presentation.** Median time to ICH: 525 days on TPV/r therapy. Hemophiliac patients: increased spontaneous bleeding tendency in joints, muscles, soft tissues, and urinary tract (hematuria).

C. **Frequency.** In 2006, 13 cases of ICH were reported with TPV/r use, including 8 fatalities. The increased frequency of bleeding in hemophilia is unknown.

D. Risk Factors. For ICH, risk factors include CNS lesions, head trauma, recent neurosurgery, coagulopathy, hypertension, alcohol abuse, anticoagulant or antiplatelet therapy.

E. Prevention/Monitoring. For ICH, avoid TPV/r in patients at risk for ICH. For bleeding in hemophiliac patients, consider using an NNRTI-based regimen and monitor for spontaneous bleeding.

F. Management. For ICH, discontinue TPV/r and manage with supportive care. For bleeding episodes in hemophiliac patients, Factor VIII products may be required.

Bone Marrow Suppression

A. Causative Agent. ZDV.

B. Clinical Presentation. Onset: Few weeks to months. Laboratory abnormalities: Anemia, neutropenia. Symptoms: Fatigue due to anemia; potential increase in bacterial infections due to neutropenia.

C. Frequency. Anemia 1.1 to 4%; neutropenia 1.8-8%.

D. Risk Factors. Advanced HIV, high-dose ZDV, pre-existing anemia or neutropenia, concomitant use of bone marrow suppressants (e.g., cotrimoxazole, ribavirin, ganciclovir), certain individuals at idiosyncratic increased risk for severe ZDV-associated anemia.

E. Prevention/Monitoring. Avoid use in patients at risk. Avoid other bone marrow suppressants if possible. Monitor CBC with differential at least every three months (more frequently in patients at risk).

F. Management. Switch to another NRTI and discontinue concomitant bone marrow suppressant if there are alternative options. Otherwise, for neutropenia, identify and treat other causes, consider treatment with filgrastim; for anemia, identify and treat other causes, consider blood transfusions/erythropoietin therapy.

Clinical Hepatitis or Asymptomatic Serum Transaminase Elevation

A. Causative Agents. All NNRTI's and PI's; most NRTI's; maraviroc.

B. Clinical Presentation. Onset: NNRTI (for NVP): two-thirds within first 12 weeks; NRTI's: over months to years; PI's: generally after weeks to months. Symptoms/findings: **NNRTI's:** asymptomatic to non-specific symptoms such as anorexia, weight loss, or fatigue. Approximately 50% of patients with NVP-associated symptomatic hepatic events present with skin rash. **NRTI's:** *ZDV, ddI, d4T* can cause hepatotoxicity associated with lactic acidosis and microvesicular or macrovesicular hepatic steatosis due to mitochondrial toxicity; *3TC, FTC,* or *tenofovir*: HBV co-infected patients may develop a severe hepatic flare when these drugs are withdrawn or when resistance develops. **PI's:** Clinical hepatitis and hepatic decompensation have been reported with TPV/RTV, but also other PI's to varying degrees. Underlying liver disease increases risk. Risk due to ritonavir is dose-related.

C. **Frequency.** Varies by agent.

D. **Risk Factors.** Hepatitis B or C coinfection, alcoholism, concomitant hepatotoxic drugs, elevated ALT/AST at baseline. For NVP-associated hepatic events, increased risk in females with pre-NVP CD4 > 250/mm^3 and males with pre-NVP CD4 > 500/mm^3.

E. **Prevention/Monitoring.** NVP: Monitor liver enzymes at baseline, 2 and 4 weeks, then monthly for first 3 months, then every 3 months. TPV/RTV: Contraindicated in patients with moderate or severe hepatic insufficiency; follow others frequently during treatment. Other agents: Monitor liver enzymes at least every 3-6 months or more frequently in patients at risk. Risk due to ritonavir is dose-related.

F. **Management.** Rule out other causes of hepatoxicity (alcoholism, viral hepatitis, chronic HBV with 3TC, FTC or TDF withdrawal, HBV resistance, etc.) For symptomatic patients: discontinue all antiretrovirals (use caution in patients with chronic HBV infection treated with 3TC, FTC and/or TDF) and other potential hepatotoxic agents. After symptoms subside and serum transaminases return to normal, construct a new antiretroviral regimen without the potential offending agent(s). With chronic HBV, consider starting entecavir if 3TC, FTC, or TDF must be discontinued. For asymptomatic patients: if ALT > 5-10 x ULN, some may consider discontinuing antiretrovirals, others may continue therapy with close monitoring. After serum transaminases return to normal, construct a new antiretroviral regimen without the potential offending agent(s). **Note:** Also see acute hepatic failure (p. 37) and NRTI-associated lactic acidosis with hepatic steatosis (p. 38).

Nephrolithiasis/Urolithiasis/Crystalluria

A. **Causative Agent.** IDV most frequent; reports with atazanavir.

B. **Clinical Presentation.** Onset: any time after beginning of therapy, especially at times of reduced fluid intake. Laboratory abnormalities: pyuria, hematuria, crystalluria; rarely a rise in serum creatinine and acute renal failure. Symptoms: flank pain and/or abdominal pain (can be severe), dysuria, frequency.

C. **Frequency.** 12.4% of nephrolithiasis reported in clinical trials (4.7-34.4%).

D. **Risk Factors.** History of nephrolithiasis, inadequate fluid intake, high peak IDV concentration, prolonged IDV exposure, use of RTV-boosted IDV.

E. **Prevention/Monitoring.** Instruct patients to drink at least 1.5-2 liters of water per day, and to increase fluid intake at first sign of darkened urine. Monitor urinalysis and serum creatinine every 3-6 months.

F. **Management.** Increase hydration, pain control. Consider switching to alternative agent or therapeutic drug monitoring if treatment option is limited. Stent placement may be required for obstructive nephrolithiasis (rare).

Nephrotoxicity

A. Causative Agents. IDV, potentially TDF.

B. Clinical Presentation. Onset: IDV: months after therapy. TDF: weeks to months after therapy. Laboratory and other findings: IDV: elevated serum creatinine, pyruria, hydronephrosis or renal atrophy. TDF: elevated serum creatinine, proteinuria, hypophosphatemia, glycosuria, hypokalemia, non-anion gap metabolic acidosis. Symptoms: IDV: asymptomatic; rare progression to end-stage renal disease. TDF: asymptomatic to signs of nephrogenic diabetes insipidus, Fanconi Syndrome.

C. Frequency. Unknown.

D. Risk Factors. History of renal disease, concomitant use of nephrotoxic drugs.

E. Prevention/Monitoring. Avoid use of other nephrotoxic drugs. Ensure adequate hydration if on IDV therapy. Monitor serum creatinine, urinalysis, serum potassium and phosphorus in patients at risk.

F. Management. Stop offending agent (generally reversible). Provide supportive care and electrolyte replacement as indicated.

Neuropathy (see pp. 118-119)

Pancreatitis

A. Causative Agents. ddI alone; ddI + d4T; ddI + hydroxyurea (HU) or ribavirin (RBV); 3TC in children.

B. Clinical Presentation. Onset: usually weeks to months. Laboratory abnormalities: increased serum amylase and lipase. Symptoms: post-prandial abdominal pain, nausea, vomiting.

C. Frequency. ddI alone: 1.7%; ddI + HU: increased by 4-5 fold; ddI + RBV, d4T, or TDF: increased frequency. 3TC in children: early trials 14-18%; later trial < 1%.

D. Risk Factors. High intracellular or serum ddI concentrations; history of pancreatitis; alcoholism; hypertriglyceridemia; use of ddI + d4T, HU, or RBV; use of ddI + TDF without ddI dose reduction.

E. Prevention/Monitoring. ddI should not be used in patients with a history of pancreatitis. Avoid concomitant use of ddI with d4T, TDF, HU or RBV. Reduce ddI dose when used with TDF. Monitoring of amylase/lipase in asymptomatic patients is generally not recommended.

F. Management. Discontinue offending agent(s). Symptomatic management of pancreatitis includes bowel rest, IV hydration, pain control, then gradual resumption of oral intake. Parenteral nutrition may be necessary in patients with recurrent symptoms upon resumption of oral intake.

Skin Rash

A. Causative Agents. NVP > EFV, DLV. Also seen with ABC, APV, f-APV, ATV, TPV/RTV, DRV/RTV. Rarely can be seen with any antiretroviral agent.

B. Clinical Presentation. Onset: within first few days to weeks after initiation of therapy. Symptoms: most rashes are mild to moderate, diffuse maculopapular rashes with or without pruritus. Immediate discontinuation of antiretrovirals is required for severe rash and for rash with fever or mucus membrane involvement. TPV/RTV: Rash can be accompanied by joint pain/stiffness, throat tightness, or generalized pruritus. Also see sections on Stevens-Johnson Syndrome (p. 40) and systemic hypersensitivity reactions (p. 40).

C. Frequency. NVP: 14.8% (1.5% severe). EFV: 26% (1% grades 3-4). DLV: 35.4% (4.4% grades 3-4). ABC: < 5% in patients without hypersensitivity reaction. APV: 20-27% (1.0% grades 3-4). f-APV: 19% (< 1% grades 3-4). ATV: 21% (< 1% severe). TPV/RTV: 14% in females and 8-10% in males in Phase 2/3 trials; 33% in females in Phase 1 study with ethinyl estradiol.

D. Risk Factors. NVP: female, Black, Asian, Hispanic. f-APV, APV, TPV (sulfonamide derivatives): potential for cross hypersensitivity with other sulfa drugs. TPV: female gender. EFV: higher incidence in children.

E. Prevention/Monitoring. NVP: always use a 2-week low-dose lead-in period. Avoid use of corticosteroid during NVP dose escalation (may increase incidence of rash). Advise patients to report first sign of rash. Most experts suggest avoidance of EFV or DLV in patients with a history of severe rash from NVP, and vice versa.

F. Management. Mild to moderate rash may be managed by symptomatic treatment with antihistamines and continuation of offending agent. Discontinue therapy if skin rash progresses to severe in nature (accompanied by blisters, fever, mucous membrane involvement, conjunctivitis, edema, or arthralgias) or in presence of systemic symptoms (including fever). **Do not restart offending agent in case of severe rash.** If rash develops during first 18 weeks of NVP treatment, obtain serum transaminases to rule out symptomatic hepatic event.

Chapter 4

Treatment Failure and Resistance Testing

ANTIRETROVIRAL TREATMENT FAILURE (Table 4.1)

Antiretroviral treatment failure can be defined in various ways. These include **virologic failure** (inability to achieve virologic suppression, or occurrence of virologic rebound), **immunologic failure** (progressive CD4 decline), and **clinical failure** (HIV disease progression). Causes of treatment failure include inadequate adherence, preexisting drug resistance, regimen complexity, side effects, and suboptimal pharmacokinetics. All of these factors can lead to persistent viral replication and evolution of drug resistance.

Regimens for treatment-experienced patients need to be individualized, with the help of resistance testing. Such testing can identify drugs that are likely to be active in patients with prior treatment failures, although other factors, such as regimen tolerability, drug-drug interactions, and achievable plasma concentrations are also important. Choosing an individualized antiretroviral regimen, optimally containing at least two fully active agents, is critical in maximizing the chances for virologic suppression.

Poor medication adherence is the most common cause of treatment failure (J Infect Dis 2005;191:339-347). With poor adherence, subinhibitory drug levels occur, allowing ongoing viral replication and often the emergence of resistant virus. Such resistant variants are likely preexisting mutants that have escaped drug control or host immune failure. The level of adherence required to prevent treatment failure varies depending on the regimen used. In the early protease inhibitor (PI) era, there was a sharp increase in failure rates when adherence fell below 95% (Ann Intern Med 2000;133:21-30). More recent analyses suggest that lower levels of adherence are required when using NNRTI-based regimens, likely due to the longer plasma half-life of nevirapine and efavirenz compared with PI's (Clin Infect Dis 2006;43:939-41). One potential limitation of this analysis for the current treatment era is that it involved unboosted PI's, which have less favorable pharmacokinetics than PI's given with low-dose ritonavir.

For patients with virologic failure due to noncompliance, the first step is to establish how much of the combination regimen is being taken. Often a patient will have stopped an entire regimen simultaneously either due to poor tolerability or psychosocial issues. In this context, virologic failure usually occurs *without* the development of antiretroviral drug resistance, as viremia occurs in the absence of selective pressure of the antivirals. Starting a new regimen (one with the goal of fewer side effects) or restarting the same regimen with a renewed emphasis on the importance of adherence may result in treatment virologic suppression.

A. Types of Treatment Failure

1. **Virologic Failure** is most strictly defined as the inability to achieve or maintain virologic suppression. In a treatment-naïve patient, the HIV RNA level should be < 400 copies/mL after 24 weeks or < 50 copies/mL by 48 weeks after starting therapy. Virologic rebound is seen when there is repeated detection of HIV RNA

after virologic suppression in either treatment-naïve or treatment-experienced patients.

2. **Immunologic Failure** can occur in the presence or absence of virologic failure and is defined as a failure to increase the CD4 cell count by 25-50 cells/mm^3 above baseline during the first year of therapy, or as a decrease in CD4 cell count to below baseline count while on therapy.
3. **Clinical Failure** is the occurrence or recurrence of HIV-related events after at least 3 months on potent antiretroviral therapy, excluding events related to an immune reconstitution syndrome.
4. **Usual Sequence of Treatment Failure.** Virologic failure usually occurs first, followed by immunologic failure, and finally by clinical progression (J Infect Dis. 2000;181:946-953). These events may be separated by months or years and may not occur in this order in all patients.

B. Goals After Virologic Failure. When patients have detectable HIV RNA on treatment, clinicians should attempt to identify the cause of their lack of response and set a treatment goal of achieving full virologic suppression (HIV RNA < 50 copies/mL). The availability of drugs from older classes with enhanced activity against resistant virus and newer agents from novel classes make this an attainable goal for virtually every treatment-experienced patient. In addition to improving clinical and immunologic outcomes, this strategy will also prevent the selection of additional resistance mutations (Ann Intern Med 2000;133:471-473; J Acquir Immune Defic Syndr 2005;40:34-40). Provided that medication adherence issues and regimen tolerability have been addressed, the regimen should be changed sooner than later.

In rare cases, achieving an undetectable HIV RNA level in patients with an extensive prior treatment history may not be possible. The main goals in these patients should be partial suppression of HIV RNA below the pretreatment baseline level, which in turn leads to the preservation of immune function and the prevention of clinical progression. A likely explanation for this phenomenon is that continued antiretroviral therapy in the face of resistance selects for less fit virus, ultimately leading to less immediate immunologic damage (J Infect Dis 2000;181:946-953; AIDS 2004;18:1539-1548). It is well documented that such patients on treatment have a slower CD4 cell decline than those not on therapy who have wild-type virus (Lancet 2004;364:51-62). Consequently, even with extensive drug resistance and virologic rebound, antiviral therapy should be continued, since stopping therapy is associated with higher rates of disease progression (J Infect Dis 2002;186:189-197; N Engl J Med 2003;349:837-846).

C. Antiretroviral Regimens After Virologic Failure

1. **Timing of Switch.** The likelihood of achieving an undetectable HIV RNA level after virologic failure is greater when treatment is changed prior to the accumulation of multiple resistance mutations. Two additional important factors influencing the outcome of subsequent treatment are the level of virologic

rebound and degree of CD4 decline (J Acquir Immune Defic Syndr 1999:22:132-138; HIV Clin Trials 2005;6:281-290). For example, in the TORO studies of enfuvirtide plus an optimized background regimen versus an optimized background regimen alone, study participants with a CD4 cell count > 100/mm^3 and/or an HIV RNA level < 100,000 copies/mL were significantly more likely to respond to therapy with or without enfuvirtide (HIV Clin Trials 2005;6:281-290). Additional predictors were exposure to 10 or fewer prior antiretrovirals and having a greater number of active drugs in the optimized background regimen.

2. **Delayed Switch Strategy.** Patients with extensive triple-class drug resistance may be clinically stable, with relatively preserved CD4 cell counts. If 2 (or preferably 3) well-tolerated and active drugs are not available, deferring a switch to preserve active drug classes reduces the risk of selecting further resistance with sequential monotherapy. This delayed switch strategy is most defensible when the CD4 cell count is in a clinically safe range (> 200/mm^3) and the patient is amenable and adherent to a strategy of regular clinical and laboratory monitoring. The risk of this approach is the selection of additional resistance mutations, which may compromise future options. Delayed switching of failing regimens should generally be avoided given the recent approval of several agents with activity against resistant viruses. If delayed switching is unavoidable, however, due to patient refusal to change therapy or other issues, providers should ensure that the regimen is less likely to select for additional resistance mutations (see "Holding" Regimens, below).
3. **"Holding" Regimens.** For patients who cannot switch therapy (adherence or financial barriers, no availability of at least 2 active agents), it is reasonable to continue a regimen chosen to maintain clinical stability – sometimes referred to as a "holding" regimen. In the face of incomplete viral suppression, holding regimens should have the following components: (1) at least 2 NRTI's, one of them 3TC or FTC; and (2) a boosted PI based on tolerability. The NRTI's seem particularly important in maintaining a low HIV RNA level in patients with incomplete viral suppression (J Infect Dis 2005;192:1537-44). There is no evidence that NNRTI's continue to exert antiviral or other benefit after resistance develops, and continuing them may select for further NNRTI mutations, limiting subsequent response to new agents in this drug class, such as etravirine. The data on continued use of enfuvirtide after virologic rebound are conflicting in this regard; our practice is generally to discontinue enfuvirtide given the requirement for twice daily injections, the high cost of the medication, and the possibility of future fusion inhibitors with a similar mechanism of action and related resistance profiles.
4. **Blips.** It is important to emphasize that transient, low-level detectable HIV RNA levels – sometimes called "blips" – are often not indicative of virologic failure. In one study, 10 patients with virologic suppression (HIV RNA < 50 copies/mL) underwent intensive analysis with 36 visits over approximately 3 months (JAMA

2005;293:817-829). Of more than 700 viral load measurements, 26 samples showed transient low-level viremia. However, blips did not predict subsequent treatment failure or indicate underlying resistance. As a result, clinicians should not act based on single viral load measurements above the limit of detection but should confirm these results before changing treatment. In contrast, patients with persistent low-level viremia (> 400 and < 1000 HIV RNA copies/mL) have exhibited increases in immune activation and a higher risk of viral resistance evolution and subsequent virologic failure (*AIDS*. 2004;18:981-989).

D. Immunologic and Clinical Failure. Most cases of immunologic and clinical failure are seen after virologic rebound, in particular in patients who have completely stopped antiretroviral therapy. However, patients who have virologic suppression will rarely experience a limited CD4 response, or even a decline. Factors variably associated with poor immunologic response include older age, hepatitis C virus coinfection, use of NNRTI- rather than PI-based therapy, use of zidovudine (which can reduce total white blood cell count), and the combination of tenofovir plus didanosine (J Infect Dis 2006;193:259-268; Clin Infect Dis 2005;41:901-905). The management of patients with poor CD4 response despite virologic suppression is not well established; our practice is to modify the antiretroviral regimen if there is a specific component known to reduce CD4 response (e.g., tenofovir + ddI, or ZDV-induced leukopenia), and to consider use of a boosted PI if the patient is on an NNRTI. Importantly, the clinical prognosis for patients with virologic responses even without substantial CD4 increases is superior to those with comparable CD4 cell counts who do not have suppression of viremia (Ann Intern Med. 2000;133:401-410). Actual clinical progression in the face of virologic suppression is rare, and often a manifestation of the immune reconstitution inflammatory syndrome (IRIS) rather than actual HIV disease progression. Such cases represent an enhanced immune response to a preexisting opportunistic process and not the acquisition of a new infection (Clin Infect Dis 2006;42:418-427). In cases of IRIS, usually the current antiretroviral therapy should be continued, with treatment of the underlying process and, if necessary, adjunctive anti-inflammatory therapy with corticosteroids.

Table 4.1. Management of Antiretroviral Treatment Failure

Type of Failure	Recommended Approach	Comments
Virologic failure *Limited or intermediate prior treatment*	Assess for adherence and regimen tolerability. Obtain genotype resistance test. Select new regimen based on resistance test results and tolerability	Usually associated with limited or no detectable resistance. If no resistance is found, consider re-testing for resistance 2-4 weeks after resuming antivirals. Stop NNRTI's if resistance is detected. Likelihood of virologic suppression is high if adherence is good
Extensive prior treatment	Assess for adherence and regimen tolerability. Obtain resistance test – consider phenotype, "virtual phenotype," or phenotype-genotype combination if level of resistance is likely to be high. Obtain viral tropism assay to assess possible use of CCR5 antagonist. Select new regimen using at least 2 new active agents; if 2 new active agents not available, continue a "holding" regimen	In patients with resistance to NRTI's, NNRTI's, and PI's, the new regimen should generally contain: (1) at least one drug from a new drug class (integrase inhibitor, CCR5 antagonist, or fusion inhibitor); (2) a boosted PI with activity against resistant viruses (tipranavir or darunavir); and (3) one or two NRTI's, one of them 3TC or FTC. A holding regimen should always contain 3TC or FTC plus a boosted PI; NNRTI's should never be used
Low-level HIV RNA (50-1000 copies)	Assess for adherence, drug-drug interactions, intercurrent illness, recent immunizations. Repeat test in 3-4 weeks	For low-level viremia followed by undetectable HIV RNA ("blip"), no treatment change is necessary. If HIV RNA is persistently detectable at > 500 copies/mL, obtain resistance test as described above, and treat accordingly. If HIV RNA is persistently detectable between 50-500 copies/mL, consider regimen "intensification" with use of an additional agent
Immunologic failure *Detectable HIV RNA*	Assess for adherence and tolerability. If non-adherent, resume treatment after barriers to adherence are addressed. If adherent, obtain resistance testing and alter therapy as described above	If HIV RNA is back to pre-treatment baseline, non-adherence is the most likely explanation
Suppressed HIV RNA	Investigate for modifiable conditions that may be associated with impaired CD4 response (chronic HCV, treatment with ZDV, TDF + ddI). If no modifiable conditions found, continue current regimen	Prognosis for patients with suppressed HIV RNA and immunologic failure better than for those with comparable CD4 cell counts and detectable viremia

Table 4.1. Management of Antiretroviral Treatment Failure (cont'd)

Type of Failure	Recommended Approach	Comments
Clinical failure *Detectable HIV RNA*	Treat OI with appropriate anti-infective therapy. Assess for antiretroviral adherence and tolerability. Send resistance test and choose new regimen based on results of test and other treatment options	OI's (IRIS excluded) most commonly occur in those not on antiretroviral therapy due to poor compliance and/or regimen tolerability
Suppressed HIV RNA	Continue current antiretrovirals. Treat OI with appropriate anti-infective therapy. If symptoms persist and IRIS is likely, use adjunctive corticosteroids	IRIS most likely when baseline CD4 cell count is low (< 200/mm^3); onset usually weeks-to-months after starting a potent regimen. IRIS been reported with virtually all OI's. True clinical progression with suppressed HIV RNA is unusual; IRIS should not be considered a sign of treatment failure

IRIS = immune reconstitution inflammatory syndrome, OI = opportunistic infection

PRINCIPLES OF RESISTANCE TESTING

HIV drug resistance most commonly occurs as a result of non-suppressive antiretroviral regimens. Less commonly, resistance occurs as a result of transmission of a resistant strain. The prevalence of drug resistance among patients with sustained viral replication is high. In a random sample of HIV-infected American adults, NRTI resistance was found in 71% of samples, PI resistance in 41%, NNRTI resistance in 25%, and triple-class resistance in 13% (AIDS 2004;18:1393-1401). Studies have demonstrated that the presence of resistance before starting a new antiretroviral regimen increases the likelihood that the regimen will fail, and that patients whose treatment is chosen with information from resistance testing have better short-term virologic outcomes than control subjects without use of resistance tests.

Resistance testing is a highly complex diagnostic strategy that for maximal effect requires both a thorough review of the patient treatment history and an understanding of the strengths and limitations of the resistance assays. Both genotypic and phenotypic criteria for resistance are under continuous evaluation and evolution. It is therefore important to consult with updated guidelines, such as those published by the International AIDS Society (see www.iasusa.org).

In a patient's resistance testing history, the occurrence of a given mutation implies that this resistance will persist even when the selective pressure for this mutation is removed and the mutation is no longer detectable by conventional resistance testing. For example, the occurrence of the M184V mutation secondary to 3TC or FTC therapy may no longer appear on resistance tests after these drugs have been stopped. However, viruses that still harbor this mutation are "archived" and will re-emerge with resumption of these agents. Although there are literally hundreds of genotypic mutations described, certain mutations or patterns of mutations are more important than others. These are discussed below.

The correlation between the presence of resistance and response to a given combination of drugs is not always absolute. For example, even when viruses harbor several primary PI resistance mutations, ritonavir-boosted PI's may retain significant antiviral effect since achievable drug levels exceed levels required for inhibition of these strains. Among the NRTI's, it is well established that 3TC (and presumably FTC) continue to reduce HIV RNA even after development of substantial in vitro resistance to these drugs. As a result of these and other factors, continuing antiretroviral therapy even after widespread antiviral drug resistance leads to a better virologic, immunologic, and clinical outcome.

TYPES OF RESISTANCE TESTING

Two types of resistance testing can be ordered: genotypic and phenotypic. Genotype tests describe mutations known to be associated with resistance to specific drugs. Phenotype tests measure the ability of individual drugs to inhibit a recombinant virus that is derived from the patient's isolate. Advantages and disadvantages of the two types of resistance tests are described in Table 4.2.

A. Genotype Testing. In most settings where resistance testing is indicated, genotype testing is preferred over phenotype testing, as a larger number of studies having validated the predictive value of genotype testing to help enhance treatment response. Genotype testing is also more easily standardized from lab-to-lab, less expensive, and has faster turnaround time.

Table 4.2. Genotype vs. Phenotype Resistance Testing

Method	Advantages	Disadvantages
Genotype testing	• Rapid turnaround (1-2 weeks) • Less expensive than phenotyping • Detection of mutations may precede phenotypic resistance • Widely available • More sensitive than phenotype for detecting mixtures of resistant and wild-type virus, especially for patients not on treatment • Two FDA-approved genotype assays (TRUGENE, ViroSeq)	• Indirect measure of resistance • Relevance of some mutations is unclear • Unable to detect minority variants (< 20-25% of viral sample) • Complex mutational patterns may be difficult to interpret • Interpretation of results variable depending on the laboratory
Phenotype testing	• Provides direct and quantitative measure of resistance • Methodology can be applied to any antiretroviral agent, including new drugs, for which genotypic correlates of resistance are unclear • Can assess interactions among mutations • Accurate with non-B HIV subtypes • May offer an estimate of the ability of resistant viruses to grow compared to wild-type strains ("replication capacity")	• Susceptibility cut-offs not standardized between assays • Clinical cut-offs not defined for some agents • Unable to detect minority variants (< 20-25% of viral sample) • Complex technology with longer turnaround (3-4 weeks) • More expensive than genotyping • Availability limited to two laboratories in USA (Monogram and Virco)

B. **Phenotype Testing.** Phenotype testing, usually in conjunction with a genotype test, may be of particular value in the following clinical scenarios: (1) occurrence of certain viral strains that make sequencing difficult for the laboratory; (2) highly complex or contradictory genotype results, especially in multiple PI-resistant cases; and (3) when used in conjunction with therapeutic drug monitoring of protease inhibitors (rarely done in the United States currently). Phenotype testing is especially useful when deciding whether to use tipranavir or darunavir, as these are the most active agents against highly PI-resistant strains. In such a setting, predicting tipranavir or darunavir activity based on genotype testing is often difficult; in contrast, clinical cutoffs are provided by phenotype testing that detail whether these drugs are fully active, partially active, or inactive virologically.

C. **Other Options for Resistance Testing.** One of the companies that performs phenotype testing (Monogram) offers a combined phenotype/genotype test, called a "Phenosense GT." This test provides the most complete representation of resistance status, with a direct correlation between detected mutations and in vitro susceptibility. The combined test has the highest cost among commercially available assays. Another company (Virco) offers a test sometimes referred to as a "virtual" phenotype. Called "VircoType HIV," this test uses standard genotype results to predict drug susceptibility based on associations of detected mutations with existing phenotypes in a database. A benefit of this approach is that it indicates which drugs have partial activity. The cost is intermediate between genotype and phenotype testing.

D. **Co-Receptor Tropism Assay.** HIV enters the CD4 cell using both the CD4 receptor and either a CCR5 receptor (R5-tropic viruses) or a CXCR4 receptor (X4-tropic viruses). R5-tropic viruses are commonly transmitted and predominate in early infection. Over time, there is a shift in virus population to those that use both receptors (dual tropic) or to a mixture of R5 and X4 viruses. The CCR5 antagonist drug maraviroc is only active against R5-tropic viruses. As a result, when considering use of this agent, a co-receptor tropism assay should be ordered. It is reasonable to consider repeating this test for patients who experience virologic failure on maraviroc.

The best available assay currently is a modification of the Monogram phenotype; results return in 3-4 weeks, and indicate whether the viral population is R5-tropic, of dual or mixed tropism (D/M), or X4-tropic. The report also provides a summary statement about whether CCR5 antagonist drugs will be active. In clinical studies of maraviroc in treatment-experienced patients, approximately 50% of patients screened had R5-tropic virus and hence were appropriate candidates for the drug. Notably, the test is not 100% sensitive for X4-using viruses; a more sensitive assay is under development.

INDICATIONS FOR AND APPROACH TO RESISTANCE TESTING

Since the introduction of resistance testing in the late–1990s, indications for resistance testing have expanded significantly (Table 4.3). A suggested approach to HIV drug resistance testing is shown in Figure 4.1.

Table 4.3. Indications for Resistance Testing

Indication	Comments
Acute or recent (<12 months) HIV infection	Primary transmission of drug-resistant virus is well documented. If a patient is being considered for treatment in this context, then treatment should be started with a boosted PI awaiting the results of the resistance test. Modification of therapy may be necessary once the results of resistance testing are available
Prior to initiation of antiretroviral therapy in established HIV infection (especially for patients infected within previous 2 years and possibly longer)	Even with established HIV disease, transmitted resistant virus may persist for years and potentially alter selection of an initial antiretroviral regimen. Pretreatment resistance testing is especially useful in communities where the likelihood of transmitted resistance ≥ 5%. Since this rate is highly variable even within a given region depending on patient demographics, many providers now perform resistance testing as part of a baseline evaluation in all newly-diagnosed HIV patients. Disease modeling studies suggest that this strategy is cost-effective (Clin Infect Dis 2005;41:1316-23). Pre-treatment resistance testing — preferably at the time of diagnosis — is now incorporated into DHHS treatment guidelines
First regimen failure (including suboptimal HIV-1 RNA response to therapy)	Such patients usually have relatively little drug resistance, generally only to the NNRTI or 3TC/FTC component of their regimen. Nevertheless, it is helpful to have documentation of this resistance prior to choosing a new regimen. Genotype testing is preferred
Multiple regimen failures	Resistance testing in the context of multiple lines of treatment failure helps determine the resistance "density" within a drug class, and whether the patient has resistance to all 3 major drug classes (NRTI, PI, NNRTI). It is particularly challenging to choose new regimens for these "triple class" treatment failures, and phenotype testing is often useful in this setting
Pregnancy (if detectable plasma HIV RNA level)	As with all patients, the goal of treatment in pregnancy is to maximize HIV RNA suppression and hence reduce the risk of perinatal transmission as much as possible

* Adapted from: Clin Infect Dis 2003;37:113-128, and DHHS Guidelines, October, 2006, www.aidsinfo.nih.gov

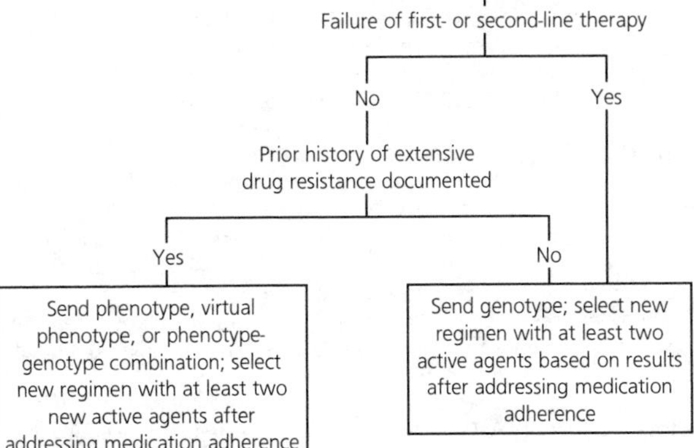
Virologic Non-Suppression Confirmed on Repeat Testing and HIV RNA Not Clearly Trending Downward
Failure of first- or second-line therapy
No
Yes
Prior history of extensive drug resistance documented
Yes
No
Send phenotype, virtual phenotype, or phenotype-genotype combination; select new regimen with at least two new active agents after addressing medication adherence
Send genotype; select new regimen with at least two active agents based on results after addressing medication adherence

Figure 4.1. Approach to HIV Drug Resistance Testing

IMPORTANT GENOTYPIC RESISTANCE PATTERNS

(see also Appendix 1: Drug Resistance Mutations in HIV-1, p. 182)

A. Nucleoside Reverse Transcriptase Inhibitors (NRTI's)

1. 3TC/FTC: M184V

- M184V emerges rapidly (days-weeks) in non-suppressive treatment regimens. This leads to a large reproducible increase in resistance of the virus to 3TC and FTC. On its own, M184V reduces the susceptibility of viruses to abacavir and ddI; however, these drugs do retain clinically significant antiviral activity even with M184V. One prospective study found that the incidence of M184V was lower in patients treated with tenofovir, FTC, and EFV than with ZDV/3TC and EFV (Gallant J, et al. International AIDS Conference, 2006, Abstract TUPE0064).
- Despite this resistance, significant antiviral activity of 3TC/FTC-containing regimens is often maintained for a prolonged period of time. Common explanations include: (1) M184V increases viral susceptibility to certain other NRTI's, notably ZDV, d4T, and tenofovir; (2) viruses with M184V have a lower replication capacity in vitro than wild-type viruses; and (3) 3TC/FTC exert an antiviral effect despite the presence of high-level phenotypic resistance.
- The combination of rapid development of resistance to 3TC/FTC, the potential benefits of the M184V mutation otherwise, and the excellent tolerability of these drugs leads to a clinical dilemma: should the drug be continued even in

the face of resistance? Our practice is typically to continue the 3TC/FTC in patients who otherwise have extensive resistance and may benefit from the reduced viral fitness imparted by the M184V mutation. Supportive data for this approach is derived from studies in which patients receiving 3TC and having M184V experienced significant increases in HIV RNA after 3TC was discontinued (Clin Infect Dis 2005;41;236-42, AIDS 2006;20:795-803).

2. **ZDV/d4T: Thymidine-Associated Mutations (TAMs)**
   - The thymidine-associated mutations are M41L, D67N, K70R, L210W, T215Y, and K219Q.
   - TAMs emerge slowly and sequentially with ZDV and d4T-containing regimens. As ZDV and d4T are combined with 3TC or FTC for initial therapy, the M184V mutation generally evolves before the occurrence of TAMs.
   - As with other non-suppressive regimens, in general the longer a patient is on an ZDV or d4T-containing regimen with a detectable HIV RNA, the greater the number of TAMs the patient will accumulate.
   - The degree of resistance to ZDV and d4T as well as other NRTI's correlates with the total number of TAMs. Only 1 or 2 TAMs may reduce susceptibility to ZDV or d4T, whereas 3 or more TAMs are required to reduced susceptibility (and virologic response) to ABC, ddI, and TDF. (Note that M184V plus only 1 TAM will reduce viral susceptibility to ABC.)
   - Often patients will evolve along one of two different TAM pathways: (1) M41L, L210W, T215Y: this occurs more commonly and is associated with broader resistance, including all other NRTI's as well as TDF; or (2) D67N, K70R, and K219Q: this induces a lower-level of resistance, and TDF treatment retains full activity.

3. **Tenofovir: K65R**
   - K65R reduces in vitro susceptibility to tenofovir, 3TC, ddI, and abacavir. In patients with prior ZDV or d4T treatment and associated TAMs, selection of K65R rarely occurs.
   - As with the TAMs described above, in a typical combination regimen using TDF, 3TC or FTC, and EFV, the first mutations to appear are M184V (selected by 3TC and FTC) and NNRTI-associated mutations. In patients with continued non-suppressive therapy, K65R may also develop.
   - The consequence of this pattern is broad NRTI resistance (analogous to multiple TAMs) and high-level NNRTI resistance (if NNRTI resistance mutations are present). Viruses harboring the K65R mutation remain susceptible to ZDV, and are sometimes "hypersusceptible," indicating that ZDV is more active vs. K65R mutants than against wild-type virus. Preliminary data suggest that patients with K65R (plus M184V and NNRTI resistance) can usually be successfully treated with salvage regimens, generally in those containing boosted PI's.
   - As with M184V, in vitro data suggest that K65R reduces replication capacity, and that both together reduce replication capacity more than either one alone.

- K65R also may develop in treatment-naïve patients placed on abacavir, ddI, or d4T-containing initial regimens. More commonly, however, d4T will select for TAMs, and ddI and abacavir for L74V.

4. **Abacavir, ddI: L74V**
   - Virologic failure of initial therapy with abacavir or ddI (plus 3TC or FTC) most commonly selects initially for the M184V mutation, followed by L74V.
   - L74V reduces susceptibility to ABC and ddI; ZDV remains fully active. The data on TDF activity are conflicting.

5. **Multinucleoside Resistance Patterns: Q151M and T69ins**
   - Before the triple-therapy era, Q151M and T69 insertion mutation pattern (T69ins) developed in patients who were on prolonged ZDV/ddI or d4T/ddI-containing regimens with virologic failure.
   - The occurrence of these mutational patterns is rare today.
   - Q151M reduces susceptibility to all NRTI's except tenofovir.
   - If the T69ins is accompanied by 1 or more TAMs, all NRTI's (including TDF) show reduced susceptibility.

B. **Non-Nucleoside Reverse Transcriptase Inhibitors (NNRTI's).** Unsuccessful treatment with NNRTI's leads rapidly to selection of NNRTI-associated resistance mutations. These mutations generally share two important properties: (1) a nearly complete loss of antiviral activity (contrast 3TC or FTC resistance); and (2) a high degree of cross-resistance between nevirapine, delavirdine, and efavirenz. As a result, sequencing of these NNRTI's after resistance develops is not possible. The most common resistance mutation selected by efavirenz is K103N, and nevirapine often selects for Y181C, except when given with ZDV. Less common mutational patterns seen with NNRTI's are L100I, V106A/M, Y181C/I, Y188L, G190S/A, and M230L. As noted above, all may reduce susceptibility to all the drugs in the class. In vitro, efavirenz retains activity against viruses that have only the Y181C mutation selected by nevirapine. As a result, genotype reports may cite efavirenz viruses with Y181C as "possibly resistant" to efavirenz. However, clinical studies suggest that efavirenz efficacy will be reduced, possibly because of the presence of primary efavirenz resistance mutations that are below the level of detection of the genotype assay.

Etravirine is the first NNRTI with documented clinical activity against some NNRTI-resistant viruses. In the DUET studies, treatment-experienced patients with documented NNRTI resistance received either etravirine or placebo; they also received an optimized background regimen containing at least DRV/r, plus other agents selected by the investigators. At 24 weeks, viral load and CD4 cell count data significantly favored etravirine over placebo (Lancet 2007;370:39-48). In this study, response to etravirine was diminished only when patients had at least three of the following mutations (which are also included in the IAS–USA set): V90I, A98G, L100I, K101E/P, V106I, V179D/F, Y181C/I/V, and G190A/S. Importantly, baseline presence of the K103N mutation — the most common mutation seen in patients with treatment failure on efavirenz — does not affect response to etravirine, nor does the presence of the single mutations Y181C or G190A.

C. Protease Inhibitors (PI's)

1. Nelfinavir: D30N

- Virologic failure on a nelfinavir-containing regimen is most commonly associated with the D30N mutation, sometimes with N88D. While conferring high-level resistance to NFV, other PI's retain activity against these viruses.
- Clinical studies have confirmed that second PI's – especially when "boosted" with ritonavir – can be used to salvage virologic failures with D30N mutations. A potential disadvantage of this strategy is that 3TC and sometimes other NRTI-based mutations are often present as well.
- A minority of treatment failures with nelfinavir will select for the L90M mutation, which is associated with broader resistance to PI's than D30N. The L90M pathway is more common in non-subtype B viruses, which are considerably more prevalent outside of the United States and Western Europe.

2. Atazanavir: I50L

- In patients without prior PI treatment, unboosted atazanavir selects for the I50L mutation, usually after selection of 3TC or other NRTI resistance. As with D30N and nelfinavir, I50L reduces susceptibility to ATV but not to other PI's.
- On phenotype testing, viruses with I50L alone often demonstrate hypersusceptibility to other PI's – that is, non-ATV PI's appear to be more active against these viruses than against wild-type strains. The clinical significance of this phenomenon is unknown, as there are no controlled studies evaluating sequencing of PI's after ATV failure.
- PI-experienced patients treated with ATV rarely select for I50L, and more typical PI-mutations emerge.
- The resistance pattern selected by boosted ATV in treatment-naive patients is thus far unknown. One study showed no PI resistance mutations or virologic rebound on boosted ATV, analogous to other boosted PI's (presented at 13th CROY, Abst. 107LB, Denver, CO, 2006).

3. Fosamprenavir: I50V

- Use of unboosted FPV may select for the I50V mutation, generally occurring (as with NFV and ATV) along with some degree of NRTI resistance.
- I50V reduces susceptibility to lopinavir, ritonavir, and darunavir; other PI's retain activity, at least as measured by phenotype testing.
- Sequencing of PI's after development of I50V or other patterns of FPV failure has not been studied in controlled trials.

4. General protease inhibitor resistance mutations: L10F/I/R/V, V32I, M46I/L, I54V/M/L, V82A/F/T/S, I84V/A/C, and L90M

- The presence of an increasing number of mutations from the above list generally confers broad PI resistance to all FDA-approved PI's.
- With < 4 mutations from the above list, ritonavir-boosted atazanavir and lopinavir had similar virologic activity; with 4 or more such mutations, lopinavir was more active (AIDS 2006;20:847-53).
- When choosing a new regimen for patients with a high degree of PI resistance,

phenotype testing is preferred. Tipranavir and darunavir are currently the PI's with the greatest activity against PI-resistant viruses. To further increase the chances of achieving virologic suppression, all tipranavir- or darunavir-treated patients should also receive, if possible, at least one other fully active drug, along with the most active (often recycled) NRTI's. In most cases currently, this other active drug will be a drug from a newer drug class, such as an integrase inhibitor, CCR5 antagonist, or fusion inhibitor. See Figure 4.2 for the recommended approach.

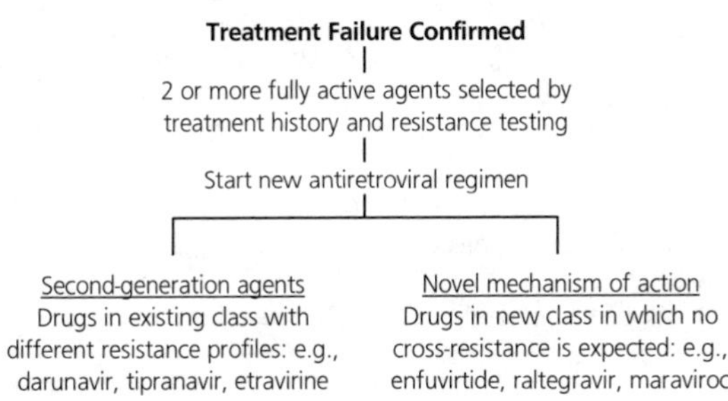
Treatment Failure Confirmed
2 or more fully active agents selected by treatment history and resistance testing
Start new antiretroviral regimen
Second-generation agents
Drugs in existing class with different resistance profiles: e.g., darunavir, tipranavir, etravirine
Novel mechanism of action
Drugs in new class in which no cross-resistance is expected: e.g., enfuvirtide, raltegravir, maraviroc

Figure 4.2. Approach to Patients with Virologic Failure and Multiclass Resistance

From: Department of Health and Human Services Panel on Antiretroviral Guidelines for Adults and Adolescents. Aidsinfo.nih.gov

Chapter 5

Prophylaxis and Treatment of Opportunistic Infections

PROPHYLAXIS OF OPPORTUNISTIC INFECTIONS

Patients with HIV disease are at risk for infectious complications not otherwise seen in immunocompetent patients. Such opportunistic infections occur in proportion to the severity of immune system dysfunction (reflected by CD4 cell count depletion). While community acquired infections (e.g., pneumococcal pneumonia) can occur at any CD4 cell count, "classic" HIV-related opportunistic infections (PCP, toxoplasmosis, cryptococcus, disseminated *M. avium* complex, CMV) do not occur until CD4 cell counts are dramatically reduced. Specifically, it is rare to encounter PCP in HIV patients with CD4 > 200/mm^3, and CMV and disseminated MAC typically occur at median CD4 < 50/mm^3. Indications for prophylaxis and specific prophylaxis regimens are summarized in Table 5.1 and detailed in Table 5.2. The U.S. Public Health Service/Infectious Diseases Society of America guidelines for the prevention of opportunistic infections in persons infected with HIV can be found at www.aidsinfo.nih.gov.

Table 5.1. Overview of Prophylaxis of Opportunistic Infections (see Table 5.2 for details)

Infection	Indication for Prophylaxis	Intervention
PCP	CD4 < 200/mm^3	TMP-SMX
TB (M. tuberculosis)	PPD > 5 mm (current or past) or contact with active case	INH
Toxoplasma	IgG Ab (+) and CD4 < 100/mm^3	TMP-SMX
MAC	CD4 < 50/mm^3	Azithromycin or clarithromycin
S. pneumoniae	CD4 > 200/mm^3	Pneumococcal vaccine
Hepatitis B	Susceptible patients	Hepatitis B vaccine
Hepatitis A	HCV (+) and HA Ab (–); HCV (–) and HA Ab (–) gay men and travelers to endemic areas, chronic liver disease	Hepatitis A vaccine
Influenza	All patients	Annual flu vaccine
VZV	Exposure to chickenpox or shingles; no prior history	VZIG

Ab = antibody; HA = Hepatitis A; HCV = Hepatitis C virus; VZIG = varicella-zoster immune globulin; VZV = varicella- zoster virus; other abbreviations (p. 3)

Table 5.2. Prophylaxis of Opportunistic Infections in HIV

Infection	Indications and Prophylaxis	Comments
P. jiroveci (carinii) pneumonia (PCP)	Indications: CD4 < 200/mm^3, oral thrush, constitutional symptoms, or previous history of PCP Preferred prophylaxis: TMP-SMX 1 DS tablet (PO) q24h or 1 SS tablet (PO) q24h. 1 DS tablet (PO) 3x/week is also effective, but daily dosing may be slightly more effective based on 1 comparative study (Clin Inf Dis 1999;29:775-83) Alternate prophylaxis: Dapsone 100 mg (PO) q24h (preferred as second-line by most; more effective than aerosolized pentamidine when CD4 cell count < 100/mm^3) **or** Atovaquone 1500 mg (PO) q24h (comparably effective to dapsone and aerosolized pentamidine; more GI toxicity vs. dapsone, but less rash) **or** Aerosolized pentamidine 300 mg via Respirgard II nebulizer once monthly (exclude active pulmonary TB first to avoid nosocomial transmission)	Without prophylaxis, 80% of AIDS patients develop PCP, and 60-70% relapse within one year after the first episode. Prophylaxis with TMP-SMX also reduces the risk for toxoplasmosis and possibly bacterial infections. Among patients with prior non-life-threatening reactions to TMP-SMX, 55% can be successfully rechallenged with 1 SS tablet daily, and 80% can be rechallenged with gradual dose escalation using TMP-SMX elixir (8 mg TMP + 40 mg SMX/mL) given as 1 mL x 3 days, then 2 mL x 3 days, then 5 mL x 3 days, then 1 SS tablet (PO) q24h. Primary and secondary prophylaxis may be discontinued if CD4 cell counts increase to > 200/mm^3 for 3 months or longer in response to antiretroviral therapy. Prophylaxis should be resumed if the CD4 cell count decreases to < 200/mm^3
Toxoplasmosis	Indications: CD4 < 100/mm^3 with positive toxoplasmosis serology (IgG) Preferred prophylaxis: TMP-SMX 1 DS tablet (PO) q24h Alternate prophylaxis: Dapsone 50 mg (PO) q24h + pyrimethamine 50 mg (PO) weekly + folinic acid 25 mg (PO) weekly **or** Dapsone 100 mg/pyrimethamine 50 mg twice weekly (no folinic acid) **or** Atovaquone 1500 mg (PO) q24h	Incidence of toxoplasmosis in seronegative patients is too low to warrant chemoprophylaxis. Primary prophylaxis can be discontinued if CD4 cell counts increase to > 200/mm^3 for at least 3 months in response to antiretroviral therapy. Secondary prophylaxis (chronic maintenance therapy) may be discontinued in patients who responded to initial therapy, remain asymptomatic, and whose CD4 counts increase to > 200/mm^3 for 6 months or longer in response to antiretroviral therapy. Prophylaxis should be restarted if the CD4 count decreases to < 200/mm^3. Some experts would obtain an MRI of the brain as part of the evaluation prior to stopping secondary prophylaxis

Table 5.2. Prophylaxis of Opportunistic Infections in HIV (cont'd)

Infection	Indications and Prophylaxis	Comments
Tuberculosis (M. tuberculosis)	Indications: PPD induration ≥ 5 mm or history of positive PPD without prior treatment, or close contact with active case of TB. Must exclude active disease with clinical assessment and chest x-ray before starting preventive therapy. Indicated at any CD4 cell count Preferred prophylaxis: INH 300 mg (PO) q24h x 9 months + pyridoxine 50 mg (PO) q24h x 9 months Alternate prophylaxis: Rifampin 600 mg (PO) q24h x 2 months + pyrazinamide 20 mg/kg (PO) q24h x 2 months. Rifampin should not be given to patients receiving PI's	Consider prophylaxis for skin test negative patients when the probability of prior TB exposure is > 10% (e.g., patients from developing countries, IV drug abusers in some cities, prisoners). However, a trial testing this strategy in the U.S. did not find a benefit for empiric prophylaxis. Rifampin plus pyrazinamide x 2 months was effective in a multinational clinical trial (but the combination may ↑ hepatotoxicity). Rifabutin may be substituted for rifampin in rifampin-containing regimens (see p. 70 for dosing)
M. avium complex (MAC)	Indications: CD4 < 50/mm^3 Preferred prophylaxis: Azithromycin 1200 mg (PO) once a week (fewest number of pills; fewest drug interactions; may add to efficacy of PCP prophylaxis) **or** Clarithromycin 500 mg (PO) q12h (more effective than rifabutin; associated with survival advantage; resistance detected in some breakthrough cases) Alternate prophylaxis: Rifabutin (less effective). See TB (p. 70) for dosing	Macrolide options (azithromycin, clarithromycin) preferable to rifabutin. Azithromycin is generally preferred, especially for patients on protease inhibitors (fewer drug interactions). Primary prophylaxis may be discontinued if CD4 cell counts increase to > 100/mm^3 and HIV RNA suppresses for 3-6 months or longer in response to antiretroviral therapy. Secondary prophylaxis may be discontinued for CD4 cell counts that increase to > 100/mm^3 x 6 months or longer in response to antiretroviral therapy if patients have completed 12 months of MAC therapy and have no evidence of disease. Resume MAC prophylaxis for CD4 < 100/mm^3
Pneumococcus *(S. pneumoniae)*	Indications: CD4 > 200/mm^3 Preferred prophylaxis: Pneumococcal polysaccharide (23 valent) vaccine.* Re-vaccinate x 1 at 5 years	Incidence of invasive pneumococcal disease is > 100-fold higher in HIV patients. Efficacy of vaccine is variable in clinical studies
Influenza	Indications: Generally recommended for all patients Preferred prophylaxis: Influenza vaccine (inactivated whole virus and split virus vaccine)*	Give annually (optimally October–January). New intranasal live virus vaccine is contraindicated in immunosuppressed patients

Table 5.2. Prophylaxis of Opportunistic Infections in HIV (cont'd)

Infection	Indications and Prophylaxis	Comments
Hepatitis B	Indications: All susceptible (anti-HBcAb negative and anti-HBsAg negative) patients Preferred prophylaxis: Hepatitis B recombinant DNA vaccine*	Response rate is lower than in HIV-negative controls. Repeat series if no response, especially if CD4 was low during initial series and is now increased. Management of patients with isolated antibody to hepatitis B core (i.e., "core alone") is not well defined
Hepatitis A	Indications: All susceptible patients who are also infected with hepatitis C; HAV-susceptible seronegative gay men or travelers to endemic areas; any chronic liver disease; illegal drug users Preferred prophylaxis: Hepatitis A vaccine*	Response rate is lower than in HIV-negative controls
Measles, mumps, rubella	Indications: Patients born after 1957 and never vaccinated; patients vaccinated between 1963-1967 Preferred prophylaxis: MMR (measles, mumps, rubella) vaccine*	Single case of vaccine-strain measles pneumonia in severely immuno-compromised adult who received MMR; vaccine is therefore contraindicated in patients with severe immunodeficiency (CD4 < 200/mm^3)
H. influenzae	Indications: Not generally recommended for adults Preferred prophylaxis: H. influenzae type B polysaccharide vaccine*	Incidence of H. influenzae disease is increased in HIV patients, but 65% are caused by non-type B strains. Unclear whether vaccine offers protection
Travel vaccines*	Indications: Travel to endemic areas	All considered safe except oral polio, yellow fever, and live oral typhoid–each a live vaccine. Most could probably be given safely to patients with high CD4 cell counts (> 350/mm^3), but data are limited

* Same dose as for normal hosts. If possible, give vaccines early in course of HIV infection, while immune system may still respond. Alternatively, to increase the likelihood of response in patients with advanced HIV disease, vaccines may be administered after 6-12 months of effective antiretroviral therapy. Vaccines should be given when patients are clinically stable, not acutely ill (e.g., give during a routine office visit, rather than during hospitalization for an opportunistic infection). Live vaccines (e.g., oral polio, oral typhoid, Yellow fever) are generally contraindicated, but measles vaccine is well-tolerated in children, and MMR vaccine is recommended for adults as described above

TREATMENT OF OPPORTUNISTIC INFECTIONS

Antiretroviral therapy (ART) and specific antimicrobial prophylaxis regimens have led to a dramatic decline in HIV-related opportunistic infections. Today, opportunistic infections occur predominantly in patients not receiving ART (due to undiagnosed HIV infection or nonacceptance of therapy), or in the period soon after starting ART (due to eliciting a previously absent inflammatory host response). Despite high rates of virologic failure in clinical practice, the rate of opportunistic infections in patients compliant with ART remains low, presumably due to continued immunologic response despite virologic failure, a phenomenon that may be linked to impaired "fitness" (virulence) of resistant HIV strains. For patients on or off ART, the absolute CD4 cell count provides the best marker of risk for opportunistic infections. Guidelines for treatment of OI's in the post-potent antiretroviral therapy era were last updated December 17, 2004 (see aidsinfo.NIH.gov.)

Respiratory Tract Opportunistic Infections

Aspergillosis, Invasive Pulmonary

Pathogen	Preferred Therapy	Alternate Therapy
Aspergillus fumigatus (rarely other species)	Voriconazole 400 mg (IV or PO) q12h x 2 days, then 200 mg (IV or PO) q12h until cured (typically 6-18 months)	Amphotericin B deoxycholate 1 mg/kg (IV) q24h until 2-3 gm total dose given (optimal duration of therapy poorly defined) **or** Amphotericin B lipid formulations (Abelcet or Ambisome) 5 mg/kg/day (IV) until cured

Clinical Presentation: Pleuritic chest pain, hemoptysis, cough in a patient with advanced HIV disease. Additional risk factors include neutropenia and use of corticosteroids
Diagnostic Considerations: Diagnosis by bronchoscopy with biopsy/culture. Open lung biopsy (usually video-assisted thorascopic surgery) is sometimes required. Radiographic appearance includes cavitation, nodules, sometimes focal consolidation. Dissemination to CNS may occur, and manifests as focal neurological deficits
Pitfalls: Positive sputum culture for Aspergillus in advanced HIV disease should heighten awareness of possible infection. Watch for drug-drug interactions between voriconazole and antiretrovirals metabolized via the cytochrome p450 system (PI's, NNRTI's)
Therapeutic Considerations: Decrease/discontinue corticosteroids, if possible. If present, treat neutropenia with granulocyte-colony stimulating factor (G-CSF) to achieve absolute neutrophil count > $1000/mm^3$. There are insufficient data to recommend chronic suppressive or maintenance therapy
Prognosis: Poor unless immune deficits can be corrected

Bacterial Pneumonia

Usual Pathogens	Preferred Therapy	Comments
Streptococcus pneumoniae (most common) *Haemophilus influenzae* *Pseudomonas aeruginosa* *Staphylococcus aureus*	**Combination therapy with** Ceftriaxone 1-2 gm (IV) q24h (or cefotaxime 1 gm [IV] q8h) ***plus*** azithromycin 500 gm q24h x 7-14 days **or monotherapy with** Levofloxacin 750 mg (PO/IV) q24h or moxifloxacin 400 mg (PO/IV) q24h x 7-14 days, depending on severity	For severe immunodeficiency (CD4 < $100/mm^3$), neutropenia, or a prior history of pseudomonas infection, broaden coverage to include *P. aeruginosa* and other gram-negative bacilli by adding **either** ceftazidime 1 gm (IV) q8h **or** cefepime 1 gm (IV) q12h **or** ciprofloxacin 750 mg (PO) q12h or 400 mg (IV) q8h. For critically-ill patients or known colonization with MRSA, add vancomycin 1 gm (IV) q12h

Clinical Presentation: HIV-infected patients with bacterial pneumonia present similar to those without HIV, with a relatively acute illness (over days) that is often associated with chills, rigors, pleuritic chest pain, and purulent sputum. Patients who have been ill over weeks to months are more likely have PCP, tuberculosis, or a fungal infection. Since bacterial pneumonia can occur at any CD4 cell count, this infection is frequently the presenting symptom of HIV disease, prompting initial HIV testing and diagnosis

Diagnostic Considerations: The most common pathogens are *Streptococcus pneumoniae*, followed by *Haemophilus influenzae*, *Pseudomonas aeruginosa*, and *Staphylococcus aureus*. The pathogens of atypical pneumonia (*Legionella pneumophila, Mycoplasma pneumoniae,* and *Chlamydia pneumoniae*) are rarely encountered, even with extensive laboratory investigation. A lobar infiltrate on chest radiography is a further predictor of bacterial pneumonia. Blood cultures should be obtained, as HIV patients have an increased rate of bacteremia compared to those without HIV

Pitfalls: Sputum gram stain and culture are generally only helpful if collected prior to starting antibiotics, and only if a single organism predominates. HIV patients with bacterial pneumonia may rarely have a more subacute opportunistic infection concurrently, such as PCP or TB

Therapeutic Considerations: Once improvement has occurred, a switch to oral therapy is generally safe. Patients with advanced HIV disease are at greater risk of bacteremic pneumonia due to gram-negative bacilli, and should be covered empirically for this condition

Prognosis: Response to therapy is generally prompt and overall prognosis is good

Pneumocystis jiroveci (carinii) Pneumonia (PCP)

Subset	Preferred Therapy	Alternate Therapy
Mild or moderate disease (pO_2 > 70 mmHg, A-a gradient < 35)	TMP-SMX DS 2 tablets (PO) q8h x 21 days	Dapsone 100 mg (PO) q24h x 21 days plus TMP 5 mg/kg (PO) q8h x 21 days (↓ leukopenia/hepatitis vs. TMP-SMX) **or** Primaquine 30 mg (PO) q24h x 21 days plus clindamycin 300-450 mg (PO) q6h-q8h x 21 days **or** Atovaquone 750 mg (PO) q12h with food x 21 days
Severe disease (pO_2 < 70 mmHg, A-a gradient > 35)	TMP/SMX (5 mg/kg TMP) (IV) q6h x 21 days **plus** Prednisone 40 mg (PO) q12h on days 1-5, then 40 mg (PO) q24h on days 6-10, then 20 mg (PO) q24h on days 11-21. Methylprednisolone (IV) can be substituted at 75% of prednisone dose	Pentamidine 4 mg/kg (IV) q24h (infused over at least 60 minutes) x 21 days plus prednisone x 21 days. (Dose reduction of pentamidine to 3 mg/kg [IV] q24h may reduce toxicity)

Clinical Presentation: Fever, cough, dyspnea; often indolent presentation. Physical exam is usually normal. Chest x-ray is variable, but commonly shows a diffuse interstitial pattern. Elevated LDH and exercise desaturation are highly suggestive of PCP

Diagnostic Considerations: Diagnosis by immunofluorescent stain of induced sputum or bronchoscopy specimen. Check ABG if O_2 saturation is abnormal or respiratory rate is increased. Serum 1, 3 beta-glucan is usually elevated and may provide additional supportive evidence for the diagnosis of PCP

Pitfalls: Slight worsening of symptoms is common after starting therapy, especially if not treated with steroids. Do not overlook superimposed bacterial pneumonia or other secondary infections, especially while on pentamidine. Patients receiving second-line agents for PCP prophylaxis—in particular aerosolized pentamidine—may present with atypical radiographic findings, including apical infiltrates, multiple small-walled cysts, pleural effusions, pneumothorax, or single/multiple nodules

Therapeutic Considerations: Outpatient therapy is possible for mild disease, but only when close follow-up is assured. Adverse reactions to TMP-SMX (rash, fever, GI symptoms, hepatitis, hyperkalemia, leukopenia, hemolytic anemia) occur in 25-50% of patients, many of whom will need a second-line regimen to complete therapy (e.g., trimethoprim-dapsone or atovaquone). Unless an adverse reaction to TMP-SMX is particularly severe (e.g., Stevens-Johnson syndrome or other life-threatening problem), TMP-SMX may be considered for PCP prophylaxis, since prophylaxis requires a much lower dose (only 10-15% of treatment dose). Patients being treated for severe PCP with TMP-SMX who do not improve after one week may be switched to pentamidine, although there are no prospective data to confirm this approach. In general, patients receiving antiretroviral therapy when PCP develops should have their treatment continued, since intermittent antiretroviral therapy can lead to drug resistance. For newly-diagnosed or antiretroviral-naive HIV patients, treatment of PCP may be completed before starting antiretroviral therapy. Steroids should be tapered (p. 69), not discontinued abruptly. Adjunctive steroids increase the risk of thrush/herpes simplex infection, but probably not CMV, TB, or disseminated fungal infection

Prognosis: Usually responds to treatment. Adverse prognostic factors include ↑ A-a gradient, hypoxemia, ↑ LDH

Pulmonary Tuberculosis (for isolates sensitive to INH and rifampin)

Pathogen	Patients NOT Receiving PI's or NNRTI's	Patients Receiving PI's or NNRTI's*
Mycobacterium tuberculosis (MTB)	Initial phase (8 weeks) INH 300 mg (PO) q24h **plus** rifampin† 600 mg (PO) q24h **plus** pyrazinamide (PZA) 25 mg/kg (PO) q24h **plus** ethambutol (EMB) 15-20 mg/kg (PO) q24h Continuation phase (18 weeks) INH 300 mg (PO) q24h **plus** rifampin† 600 mg (PO) q24h	Initial phase (8 weeks) INH 300 mg (PO) q24h **plus** rifabutin* **plus** PZA 25 mg/kg (PO) q24h **plus** EMB 15 mg/kg (PO) q24h x 8 weeks. Continuation phase (18 weeks) INH 300 mg (PO) q24h **plus** rifabutin*

* *Rifabutin dose: If PI is nelfinavir, indinavir, amprenavir or fosamprenavir, then rifabutin dose is 150 mg (PO) q24h. If PI is ritonavir, lopinavir/ritonavir or atazanavir, then rifabutin dose is 150 mg (PO) 2-3 times weekly. If NNRTI is efavirenz, then rifabutin dose is 450 mg (PO) q24h or 600 mg (PO) 2-3 times weekly. If NNRTI is nevirapine, then rifabutin dose is 300 mg (PO) q24h. Rifabutin is* ***contraindicated*** *in patients receiving delavirdine or hard-gel saquinavir. Patients receiving PI's AND NNRTI's: as above, except adjust rifabutin to 300 mg (PO) q24h.*

† *For patients receiving triple NRTI regimens, substitute rifabutin 300 mg (PO) q24h for rifampin*

Clinical Presentation: May present atypically. HIV patients with high (> 500/mm^3) CD4 cell counts are more likely to have a typical pulmonary presentation, but patients with advanced HIV disease may have a diffuse interstitial pattern, hilar adenopathy, or a normal chest x-ray. Tuberculin skin testing (TST) is helpful if positive, but unreliable if negative due to anergy

Diagnostic Considerations: In many urban areas, TB is one of the most common HIV-related respiratory illnesses. In other areas, HIV-related TB occurs infrequently except in immigrants or patients arriving from highly TB endemic areas. Maintain a high Index of suspicion for TB in HIV patients with unexplained fevers/pulmonary infiltrates

Pitfalls: Extrapulmonary and pulmonary TB often coexist, especially in advanced HIV disease

Therapeutic Considerations: Treatment by directly observed therapy (DOT) is strongly recommended for all HIV patients. If patients have cavitary disease or either positive sputum cultures or lack of clinical response at 2 months, total duration of therapy should be increased up to 9 months. If hepatic transaminases are elevated (AST > 3 times normal) before treatment initiation, treatment options include: (1) standard therapy with frequent monitoring; (2) rifamycin (rifampin or rifabutin) + EMB + PZA for 6 months; or (3) INH + rifamycin + EMB for 2 months, then INH + rifamycin for 7 months. Once-weekly rifapentine is not recommended for HIV patients. Non-severe immune reconstitution inflammatory syndrome (IRIS) may be treated with nonsteroidal anti-inflammatory drugs (NSAIDs); severe cases should be treated with corticosteroids. In all cases of IRIS, antiretroviral therapy should be continued if possible. Monitor carefully for signs of rifabutin drug toxicity (arthralgias, uveitis, leukopenia)

Prognosis: Usually responds to treatment. Relapse rates are related to the degree of immunosuppression and local risk of re-exposure to TB

CNS Opportunistic Infections

CMV Encephalitis (or Polyradiculitis)

Pathogen	Preferred Therapy	Alternate Therapy
Cytomegalovirus	Acute therapy Ganciclovir (GCV) 5 mg/kg (IV) q12h until symptomatic improvement (typically > 3 weeks). *For severe cases,* consider acute therapy with Ganciclovir 5 mg/kg (IV) q12h plus Foscarnet 60 mg/kg (IV) q8h or 90 mg/kg (IV) q12h until symptomatic improvement Follow with lifelong suppressive therapy Valganciclovir 900 mg (PO) q24h	Acute therapy Foscarnet 60 mg/kg (IV) q8h or 90 mg/kg (IV) q12h x 3 weeks Follow with lifelong suppressive therapy Valganciclovir 900 mg (PO) q24h

Clinical Presentation: Encephalitis presents as fever, mental status changes, and headache evolving over 1-2 weeks. True meningismus is rare. CMV encephalitis occurs in advanced HIV disease (CD4 < 50/mm^3), often in patients with prior CMV retinitis. Polyradiculitis presents as rapidly evolving weakness/sensory disturbances in the lower extremities, often with bladder/bowel incontinence. Anesthesia in "saddle distribution" with ↓ sphincter tone possible

Diagnostic Considerations: CSF may show lymphocytic or neutrophilic pleocytosis; glucose is often decreased. For CMV encephalitis, characteristic findings on brain MRI include confluent periventricular abnormalities with variable degrees of enhancement. Diagnosis is confirmed by CSF CMV PCR (preferred), CMV culture, or brain biopsy

Pitfalls: For CMV encephalitis, a wide spectrum of radiographic findings are possible, including mass lesions (rare). Obtain ophthalmologic evaluation to exclude active retinitis. For polyradiculitis, obtain sagittal MRI of the spinal cord to exclude mass lesions, and CSF cytology to exclude lymphomatous involvement (can cause similar symptoms)

Therapeutic Considerations: Ganciclovir plus foscarnet may be beneficial as initial therapy for severe cases. Consider discontinuation of valganciclovir maintenance therapy if CD4 increases to > 100-150/mm^3 x 6 months or longer in response to antiretroviral therapy

Prognosis: Unless immune reconstitution occurs, response to therapy is usually transient, followed by progression of symptoms

Comments: Unless CD4 cell count increases in response to antiretroviral therapy, response to anti-CMV treatment is usually transient, followed by progression of symptoms

Cryptococcal Meningitis

Pathogen	Preferred Therapy	Alternate Therapy
Cryptococcus neoformans	Acute infection (induction therapy) Amphotericin B deoxycholate 0.7 mg/kg (IV) q24h x 2 weeks ± flucytosine (5-FC) 25 mg/kg (PO) q6h x 2 weeks **or** Amphotericin B lipid formulation 4-6 mg/kg (IV) q24h x 2 weeks ± flucytosine (5-FC) 25 mg/kg (PO) q6h x 2 weeks Consolidation therapy Fluconazole 400 mg (PO) q24h x 8 weeks or until CSF cultures are sterile Chronic maintenance therapy (secondary prophylaxis) Fluconazole 200 mg (PO) q24h	Acute infection (induction therapy) Amphotericin B 0.7 mg/kg/day (IV) x 2 weeks **or** Fluconazole 400-800 mg (IV or PO) q24h x 6 weeks (less severe disease) **or** Fluconazole 400-800 mg (IV or PO) q24h plus flucytosine (5-FC) 25 mg/kg (PO) q6h x 4-6 weeks Consolidation therapy Itraconazole 200 mg (PO) q12h x 8 weeks or until CSF cultures are sterile Chronic maintenance therapy Itraconazole 200 mg (PO) q24h for intolerance to fluconazole or failed fluconazole therapy

Clinical Presentation: Often indolent onset of fever, headache, subtle cognitive deficits. Occasional meningeal signs and focal neurologic findings, though non-specific presentation is most common

Diagnostic Considerations: Diagnosis usually by cryptococcal antigen; India ink stain of CSF is less sensitive. Diagnosis is essentially excluded with a negative serum cryptococcal antigen (sensitivity of test in AIDS patients approaches 100%). If serum cryptococcal antigen is positive, CSF antigen may be negative in disseminated disease without spread to CNS/meninges. Brain imaging is often normal, but CSF analysis is usually abnormal with a markedly elevated opening pressure

Pitfalls: Be sure to obtain a CSF opening pressure, since reduction of increased intracranial pressure is critical for successful treatment. Remove sufficient CSF during the initial lumbar puncture (LP) to reduce closing pressure to < 200 mm H_20 or 50% of opening pressure. Increased intracranial pressure requires repeat daily lumbar punctures until CSF pressure stabilizes; persistently elevated pressure should prompt placement of a lumbar drain or ventriculo-peritoneal shunting. Adjunctive corticosteroids are not recommended

Therapeutic Considerations: Optimal total dose/duration of amphotericin B prior to fluconazole switch is unknown (2-3 weeks is reasonable if patient is doing well). Treatment with 5-FC is optional; however, since 5-FC is associated with more rapid sterilization of CSF, it is reasonable to start 5-FC and then discontinue it if necessary for toxicity (neutropenia, nausea). Fluconazole is preferred over itraconazole for life-long maintenance therapy. Consider discontinuation of chronic maintenance therapy in patients who remain asymptomatic with CD4 >100-200/mm^3 for > 6 months due to ART
Prognosis: Variable. Mortality up to 40%. Adverse prognostic factors include increased intracranial pressure, abnormal mental status

Progressive Multifocal Encephalopathy (PML)

Pathogen	Therapy
Reactivation of latent papovavirus (JC strain most common)	Effective antiretroviral therapy with immune reconstitution

Clinical Presentation: Hemiparesis, ataxia, aphasia, other focal neurologic defects, which may progress over weeks to months. Usually alert without headache or seizures on presentation
Diagnostic Considerations: Demyelinating disease caused by reactivation of latent papovavirus (JC strain most common). Diagnosis by clinical presentation and MRI showing patchy demyelination of white matter ± cerebellum/brainstem. JC virus PCR of CSF is useful for non-invasive diagnosis. In confusing or atypical presentation, biopsy may be needed to distinguish PML from other opportunistic infections, CNS lymphoma, or HIV encephalitis/encephalopathy
Pitfalls: Primary HIV-related encephalopathy has a similar appearance on MRI
Therapeutic Considerations: Most effective therapy is antiretroviral therapy with immune reconstitution. Some patients experience worsening neurologic symptoms once ART is initiated due to immune reconstitution induced inflammation. ART should be continued, with consideration of adjunctive steroids. Randomized controlled trials have evaluated cidofovir and vidarabine – neither is effective nor recommended
Prognosis: Rapid progression of neurologic deficits over weeks to months is common. Best chance for survival is immune reconstitution in response to antiretroviral therapy, although some patients will have progressive disease despite immune recovery

Toxoplasma Encephalitis

Pathogen	Preferred Therapy	Alternate Therapy
Toxoplasma gondii	Acute therapy (x 6-8 weeks until good clinical response) Pyrimethamine 200 mg (PO) x 1 dose, then 50 mg (< 60 kg body weight) or 75 mg (> 60 kg) (PO) q24h **plus** Sulfadiazine 1000 mg (< 60 kg) or 1500 mg (> 60 kg) (PO) q6h **plus** Leucovorin 10 mg (PO) q24h. *For severely ill patients who cannot take oral medications*, treat with TMP-SMX (5 mg/kg TMP and 25 mg/kg SMX) (IV) q12h Follow with lifelong suppressive therapy Sulfadiazine 0.5-1 gm (PO) q6h **plus** Pyrimethamine 50 mg (PO) q24h **plus** Leucovorin 10 mg (PO) q24h	Acute therapy (x 6-8 weeks until good clinical response) Pyrimethamine 200 mg (PO) x 1 dose, then 50 mg (< 60 kg body weight) or 75 mg (> 60 kg) (PO) q24h plus clindamycin 600 mg (IV or PO) q6h plus leucovorin 10 mg (PO) q24h **or** TMP-SMX (5 mg/kg TMP and 25 mg/kg SMX) (IV or PO) q12h **or** Atovaquone 1.5 gm (PO) q12h (with meals or nutritional supplement) plus pyrimethamine (as above) **or** Atovaquone 1.5 gm (PO) q12h (with meals or nutritional supplement) plus sulfadiazine 1.0-1.5 mg (PO) q6h **or** Atovaquone 1.5 gm (PO) q12h (with meals) **or** Pyrimethamine (see above) plus leucovorin 10 mg (PO) q24h plus azithromycin 900-1200 mg (PO) q24h Lifelong suppressive therapy Clindamycin 300-450 mg (PO) q6-8h plus pyrimethamine 50 mg (PO) q24h plus leucovorin 10 mg (PO) q24h (2nd choice regimen) **or** Atovaquone 750 mg (PO) q12h ± pyrimethamine 25 mg (PO) q24h and leucovorin 10 mg (PO) q24h (3rd choice regimen)

Clinical Presentation: Wide spectrum of neurologic symptoms, including sensorimotor deficits, seizures, confusion, ataxia. Fever/headache are common

Diagnostic Considerations: Diagnosis by characteristic radiographic appearance and response to empiric therapy in a for *T. gondii* seropositive patient

Pitfalls: Use leucovorin (folinic acid) 10 mg (PO) daily with pyrimethamine-containing regimens, not folate/folic acid. Radiographic improvement may lag behind clinical response

Therapeutic Considerations: Alternate agents include atovaquone, azithromycin, clarithromycin, minocycline (all with pyrimethamine if possible). Decadron 4 mg (PO or IV) q6h is useful for edema/mass effect. Chronic suppressive therapy can be discontinued if patients

are free from signs and symptoms of disease and have a CD4 cell count > 200/mm^3 for > 6 months due to ART
Prognosis: Usually responds to treatment if able to tolerate drugs. Clinical response is evident by 1 week in 70%, by 2 weeks in 90%. Radiographic improvement is usually apparent by 2 weeks. Neurologic recovery is variable

Gastrointestinal Tract Opportunistic Infections

Campylobacter Enteritis *(C. jejuni)*

Subset	Preferred Therapy
Mild disease	Might withhold therapy unless symptoms persist for several days
Moderate disease	Ciprofloxacin 500 mg (PO) q12h x 1 week **or** Azithromycin 500 mg (PO) q24h x 1 week
Bacteremia	Ciprofloxacin 500 mg (PO) q12h x 2 weeks* **or** Azithromycin 500 mg (PO) q24h x 2 weeks*

* *Consider addition of aminoglycoside in bacteremic patients*

Clinical Presentation: Acute onset of diarrhea, sometimes bloody; constitutional symptoms may be prominent
Diagnostic Considerations: Diagnosis by stool culture; bacteremia may rarely occur, so blood cultures also indicated. Suspect campylobacter in AIDS patient with diarrhea and curved gram-negative rods in blood culture. Non-jejuni species may be more strongly correlated with bacteremia
Therapeutic Considerations: Optimal therapy not well defined. Treat with quinolone or azithromycin; modify therapy based on susceptibility testing. Quinolone resistance can occur and correlates with treatment failure. Imipenem is sometimes used for bacteremia
Prognosis: Depends on underlying immune status; prognosis is generally good

Clostridium difficile Diarrhea/Colitis

Pathogen	Preferred Therapy	Alternate Therapy
C. difficile	Metronidazole 500 mg (PO) q8h x 10-14 days. Avoid use of other antibacterials if possible	Vancomycin 125 mg (PO) q6h x 10-14 days. Avoid use of other antibacterials if possible

Clinical Presentation: Diarrhea and abdominal pain following antibiotic therapy. Diarrhea may be watery or bloody. Proton pump inhibitors increase the risk. Among antibiotics, clindamycin, quinolones, and beta-lactams are most frequent. Rarely due to aminoglycosides, linezolid, doxycycline, TMP-SMX, carbapenems, daptomycin, vancomycin
Diagnostic Considerations: Most common cause of bacterial diarrhea in U.S. among HIV patients (Clin Infect Dis 2005;41:1620-7). Watery diarrhea with positive *C. difficile* toxin in stool specimen. *C. difficile* stool toxin test is sufficiently sensitive/specific. If positive, no need to

retest until negative (endpoint is end of diarrhea); if negative, no need to retest (repeat tests) will be negative). *C. difficile* colitis may be distinguished clinically from *C. difficile* diarrhea by temperature > 102°F, ↑ WBC, ↑ ESR, and/or abdominal pain. *C. difficile* virulent epidemic strain is type B1 (toxinotype III), which produces 20-times the amount of toxin A/B compared to less virulent strains

Pitfalls: In a patient with *C. difficile* diarrhea, *C. difficile* colitis is suggested by the presence of ↑ WBC, ↑ ESR, abdominal pain and temperature > 102°F; confirm diagnosis with CT of abdomen, which will show colonic wall thickening. *C. difficile* toxin may remain positive in stools for weeks following treatment; do not treat positive stool toxin unless patient has symptoms

Therapeutic Considerations: Initiate therapy for mild disease with metronidazole; symptoms usually begin to improve within 2-3 days. For moderate or severe disease, or with evidence of colitis clinically (leukocytosis, fever, colonic thickening on CT scan), vancomycin has become the preferred agent in many centers due to concern for the more virulent strain, and based on the results of some studies suggesting vancomycin is more effective. The duration of therapy should be extended beyond 14 days if other systemic antibiotics must be continued. Relapse occurs in 10-25% of patients, and rates may be higher in patients with HIV due to the frequent need for other antimicrobial therapy. First relapses can be treated with a repeat of the initial regimen of metronidazole or vancomycin. For multiple relapses, a long-term taper of vancomycin is appropriate: week 1, give 125 mg 4x/day; week 2, give 125 mg 2x/day; week 3 , give 125 mg once daily; week 4, give 125 mg every other day; weeks 5 and 6, give 125 mg every three days. Every effort should be made to resume a normal diet and to avoid other antibacterial therapies. Probiotic treatments (such as lactobacillus or *Saccharomyces boulardii*) have not yet been shown to reduce the risk of relapse in controlled clinical trials

Prognosis: Prognosis with *C. difficile* colitis is related to severity of the colitis

CMV Esophagitis/Colitis

Infection	Preferred Therapy	Alternate Therapy
Initial infection	Ganciclovir 5 mg/kg (IV) q12h x 3-4 weeks or until signs and symptoms have resolved. Valganciclovir 900 mg (PO) q12h can be used if able to tolerate oral intake. Maintenance therapy is generally not necessary but should be considered after relapses	Foscarnet 60 mg/kg (IV) q8h or 90 mg/kg (IV) q12h x 3-4 weeks or until signs and symptoms have resolved
Relapses	Valganciclovir 900 mg (PO) q24h indefinitely; consider discontinuation if CD4 > 200/mm^3 for ≥ 6 months on ART	

Clinical Presentation: Localizing symptoms, including odynophagia, abdominal pain, diarrhea, sometimes bloody stools

Diagnostic Considerations: Diagnosis by finding CMV inclusions on biopsy. CMV can affect the entire GI tract, resulting in oral/esophageal ulcers, gastritis, and colitis (most common). CMV colitis varies greatly in severity, but typically causes fever, abdominal cramping, and sometimes bloody stools

Pitfalls: CMV colitis may cause colonic perforation and should be considered in any AIDS patient presenting with an acute abdomen, especially if radiography demonstrates free intraperitoneal air

Therapeutic Considerations: Duration of therapy is dependent on clinical response, typically

3-4 weeks. Consider chronic suppressive therapy for recurrent disease. Screen for CMV retinitis
Prognosis: Relapse rate is greatly reduced with immune reconstitution due to antiretroviral therapy

Cryptosporidia Enteritis

Pathogen	Preferred Therapy	Alternate Therapy
Cryptosporidium sp.	Effective ART with immune reconstitution to CD4 > 100/mm^3 can result in complete resolution of symptoms and clearance of infection	Nitazoxanide 500 mg (PO) q12h x 4-6 weeks **or** Paromomycin 1 gm (PO) q12h x 2-4 weeks

Clinical Presentation: High-volume watery diarrhea with weight loss and electrolyte disturbances, especially in advanced HIV disease
Diagnostic Considerations: Spore-forming protozoa. Diagnosis by AFB smear of stool demonstrating characteristic oocyte. Malabsorption may occur
Pitfalls: No fecal leukocytes; organisms are not visualized on standard ova and parasite exams (need to request special stains)
Therapeutic Considerations: Anecdotal reports of antimicrobial success. Nitazoxanide may be effective in some settings, but no increase in cure rate for nitazoxanide if CD4 < 50/mm^3. Immune reconstitution in response to antiretroviral therapy is the most effective therapy, and may induce prolonged remissions and cure. Anti-diarrheal agents (Lomotil, Pepto-Bismol) are useful to control symptoms. Hyperalimentation may be required for severe cases
Prognosis: Related to degree of immunosuppression/response to antiretroviral therapy

Isospora Enteritis *(Isospora belli)*

Subset	Preferred Therapy	Alternate Therapy
Acute infection	TMP 160 mg and SMX 800 mg (IV or PO) q6h x 10 days **or** TMP 320 mg and SMX 1600 mg (IV or PO) q12h x 10-14 days	Pyrimethamine 50-75 mg (PO) q24h *plus* leucovorin 5-10 mg (PO) q24h **or** Ciprofloxacin 500 mg (PO) q12h or other fluoroquinolones
Chronic maintenance therapy for CD4 < 200 (secondary prophylaxis)	TMP 320 mg plus SMX 1600 mg (PO) q24h*	Pyrimethamine 25 mg (PO) q24h *plus* leucovorin 5-10 mg (PO) q24h*

* *Discontinuation of secondary prophylaxis may be considered if CD4 > 200/mm^3 for > 3 months*

Clinical Presentation: Severe chronic diarrhea without fever/fecal leukocytes
Diagnostic Considerations: Spore-forming protozoa *(Isospora belli)*. Oocyst on AFB smear of stool larger that cryptosporidium (20-30 microns vs. 4-6 microns). More common in HIV patients from tropical areas. Less common than cryptosporidium or microsporidia. Malabsorption may occur

Pitfalls: Multiple relapses are possible
Therapeutic Considerations: Chronic suppressive therapy may be required if CD4 cell count does not increase
Prognosis: Related to degree of immunosuppression/response to antiretroviral therapy
Comments: Immune reconstitution with ART results in fewer relapses

Microsporidia Enteritis

Pathogen	Therapy*
Microsporidia other than Enterocytozoon bienuesi	Albendazole 400 mg (PO) q12h (continue until CD4 > $200/mm^3$)
Enterocytozoon bienuesi	Fumagillin 60 mg (PO) q24h (not available in the U.S)
Trachipleistophora or Brachiola	Itraconazole 400 mg (PO) q24h plus albendazole 400 mg (PO) q12h

* *Regardless of species, ART with immune reconstitution is a critical component of treatment*

Clinical Presentation: Intermittent chronic diarrhea without fever/fecal leukocytes
Diagnostic Considerations: Spore-forming protozoa *(S. intestinalis, E. bieneusi)*. Diagnosis by modified trichrome or fluorescent antibody stain of stool. Microsporidia can rarely disseminate to sinuses/cornea. Severe malabsorption may occur
Pitfalls: Microsporidia cannot be detected by routine microscopic examination of stool due to small size
Therapeutic Considerations: Albendazole is less effective for E. bieneusi than S. intestinalis, but speciation is usually not possible. Consider treatment discontinuation for CD4 > $200/mm^3$ if patient remains asymptomatic (no signs or symptoms of microsporidiosis). If ocular infection is present, continue treatment indefinitely
Prognosis: Related to degree of immunosuppression/response to antiretroviral therapy

Oropharyngeal/Esophageal Candidiasis

Infection	Therapy	Fluconazole-Resistance
Oropharyngeal candidiasis (thrush)	Preferred therapy Fluconazole 100 mg (PO) q24h x 1-2 weeks Alternate therapy Itraconazole oral solution 200 mg (PO) q24h x 1-2 weeks **or** clotrimazole troches 10 mg (PO) 5x/day x 1-2 weeks **or** nystatin suspension 4–6 mL q6h or 1–2 flavored pastilles 4–5x/day x 1-2 weeks	Fluconazole at doses up to 800 mg (PO) q24h x 1-2 weeks **or** Caspofungin 70 mg (IV) on day 1, then 50 mg (IV) q24h x 1-2 weeks **or** Micafugin 150 mg (IV) q24h x 1-2 weeks **or** Amphotericin B 0.3 mg/kg (IV) q24h x 1-2 weeks **or** Amphotericin liposomal or lipid complex 3-5 mg/kg (IV) q24h x 1-2 weeks
Esophageal candidiasis	Preferred therapy Fluconazole 100 mg (up to 400 mg) (IV or PO) q24h x 1-2 weeks Alternate therapy Itraconazole oral solution 200 mg (PO) q24h x 2-3 weeks **or** voriconazole 200 mg (PO) q24h x 2-3 weeks **or** caspofungin 50 mg (IV) q24h x 2-3 weeks	

Oral Thrush (Candida)

Clinical Presentation: Dysphagia/odynophagia. More common/severe in advanced HIV disease
Diagnostic Considerations: Pseudomembranous (most common), erythematous, and hyperplastic (leukoplakia) forms. Pseudomembranes (white plaques on inflamed base) on buccal muscosa/tongue/gingiva/palate scrape off easily, hyperplastic lesions do not. Diagnosis by clinical appearance ± KOH/gram stain of scraping showing yeast/pseudomycelia. Other oral lesions in AIDS patients include herpes simplex, aphthous ulcers, Kaposi's sarcoma, oral hairy leukoplakia
Pitfalls: Patients may be asymptomatic
Therapeutic Considerations: Fluconazole is superior to topical therapy in preventing relapses of thrush and treating Candida esophagitis. Continuous treatment with fluconazole may lead to fluconazole-resistance, which is best treated initially with itraconazole suspension and, if no response, with IV caspofungin (or other echinocandin) or amphotericin. Chronic suppressive therapy is usually only considered for severely immunosuppressed patients
Prognosis: Improvement in symptoms are often seen within 24-48 hours

Candida Esophagitis

Clinical Presentation: Dysphagia/odynophagia, almost always in the setting of oropharyngeal thrush. Fever is uncommon
Diagnostic Considerations: Most common cause of esophagitis in HIV disease. For persistent symptoms despite therapy, endoscopy with biopsy/culture is recommended to confirm diagnosis and assess azole-resistance
Pitfalls: May extend into stomach. Other common causes of esophagitis include CMV, herpes simplex, and aphthous ulcers. Rarely, Kaposi's sarcoma, non-Hodgkin's lymphoma, zidovudine,

dideoxycytidine, and other infections may cause esophageal symptoms
Therapeutic Considerations: Systemic therapy is preferred over topical therapy. Failure to improve on empiric therapy mandates endoscopy to look for other causes, especially herpes viruses/aphthous ulcers. Consider maintenance therapy with fluconazole for frequent relapses, although the risk of fluconazole resistance is increased. Fluconazole-resistance is best treated initially with itraconazole suspension and, if no response, with IV caspofungin, micafungin, or amphotericin
Prognosis: Relapse rate related to degree of immunosuppression

Salmonella Gastroenteritis (non-typhi)

Subset	Preferred Therapy	Alternate Therapy
Mild disease	Ciprofloxacin 750 mg (PO) q12h x 1-2 weeks	TMP-SMX 1 DS (PO) q12h x 2 weeks **or** Ceftriaxone 2 gm (IV) q24h x 2 weeks **or** Cefotaxime 1 gm (IV) q8h x 2 weeks
CD4 < 200	Ciprofloxacin 750 mg (PO) q12h x 4-6 weeks	
Bacteremia	Ciprofloxacin 750 mg (PO) q12h x 4-6 weeks, then 500 mg (PO) q12h indefinitely	

Clinical Presentation: Patients with HIV are at markedly increased risk of developing salmonellosis. Three different presentations may be seen: (1) self-limited gastroenteritis, as typically seen in immunocompetent hosts; (2) a more severe and prolonged diarrheal disease, associated with fever, bloody diarrhea, and weight loss; or (3) Salmonella septicemia, which may present with or without gastrointestinal symptoms
Diagnostic Considerations: The diagnosis is established through cultures of stool and blood. Given the high rate of bacteremia associated with Salmonella gastroenteritis–especially in advanced HIV disease–blood cultures should be obtained in any HIV patient presenting with diarrhea and fever
Pitfalls: A distinctive feature of salmonella bacteremia in patients with AIDS is its propensity for relapse (rate > 20%)
Therapeutic Considerations: The mainstay of treatment is a fluoroquinolone; greatest experience is with ciprofloxacin, but newer quinolones (moxifloxacin, levofloxacin) may also be effective. For uncomplicated salmonellosis in an HIV patient with CD4 > 200/mm^3, 1-2 weeks of treatment is reasonable to reduce the risk of extraintestinal spread. For patients with advanced HIV disease (CD4 < 200/mm^3) or who have salmonella bacteremia, at least 4-6 weeks of treatment is required. Chronic suppressive therapy, given for several months or until antiretroviral therapy-induced immune reconstitution ensues, is indicated for patients who relapse after cessation of therapy. Consider using ZDV as part of the antiretroviral regimen (ZDV is active against Salmonella)
Prognosis: Usually responds well to treatment. Relapse rate in AIDS patients with bacteremia is > 20%

Shigella Enteritis *(Shigella* sp.*)*

Subset	Preferred Therapy	Alternate Therapy
No bacteremia	Fluoroquinolone (IV or PO) x 3–7 days	TMP-SMX 1 DS tablet (PO) q12h x 3-7 days **or** Azithromycin 500 mg (PO) on day 1, then 250 mg (PO) q24h x 4 days
Bacteremia	Extend treatment duration to 14 days	Extend treatment duration to 14 days

Clinical Presentation: Acute onset of bloody diarrhea/mucus
Diagnostic Considerations: Diagnosis by demonstrating organism in stool specimens. Shigella ulcers in colon are linear, serpiginous, and rarely lead to perforation. More common in gay men
Therapeutic Considerations: Shigella dysentery is more acute/fulminating than amebic dysentery. Shigella has no carrier state, unlike Entamoeba. Shigella infections acquired outside of United States have high rates of TMP-SMX resistance. Therapy is indicated to shorten the duration of illness and to prevent spread of infection. Shigella has no carrier state
Prognosis: Good if treated early. Severity of illness related to Shigella species: *S. dysenteriae* (most severe) > *S. flexneri* > *S. boydii/S. sonnei* (mildest)

Other Opportunistic Infections

Bartonella Infections *(Bartonella henselae/quintana)*

Subset	Preferred Therapy	Alternate Therapy
Non-CNS infection (bacillary angiomatosis, peliosis hepatis)	Erythromycin 500 mg (PO or IV) q6h for at least 3 months **or** Doxycycline 100 mg (IV or PO) q12h for at least 3 months	Azithromycin 600 mg (PO) q24h for at least 3 months **or** Clarithromycin 500 mg (PO) q12h for at least 3 months
CNS infection	Doxycycline 100 mg (IV or PO) q12h for at least 3 months	Azithromycin 600 mg (PO) q24h for at least 3 months **or** Clarithromycin 500 mg (PO) q12h for at least 3 months

Clinical Presentation: Skin lesions resemble Kaposi's sarcoma. CT of liver shows hepatomegaly and hypodense lesions. Bartonella can rarely present as a CNS mass lesion, similar to toxoplasmosis
Diagnostic Considerations: Diagnosis by demonstrating organism by stain/culture of skin lesions or by blood culture after lysis-centrifugation
Pitfalls: Requires life-long suppressive therapy. Does not grow in routine cultures
Therapeutic Considerations: Fluoroquinolones have variable activity in case reports and in vitro; may be considered as alternative therapy. Azithromycin likely to be better tolerated than erythromycin with fewer drug-drug interactions. Long-term suppressive therapy may be

considered in patients with relapse or reinfection
Prognosis: Related to extent of infection/degree of immunosuppression

Candida Vaginitis

Pathogen	Therapy
Candida albicans	Intravaginal miconazole suppository 200 mg q24h x 3 days or miconazole 3% x 7 days **or** Nystatin vaginal tablet 100,000U q24h x 14 days **or** Itraconazole 200 mg (PO) q12h x 1 day (or 200 mg q24h x 3 days) **or** Fluconazole 150 mg (PO) x 1 dose

Clinical Presentation: White, cheesy, vaginal discharge or vulvar rash ± itching/pain. Local infection not a sign of disseminated disease
Diagnostic Considerations: Local infection. Not a manifestation of disseminated disease
Pitfalls: Women with advanced AIDS receiving fluconazole may develop fluconazole-resistant Candida
Therapeutic Considerations: For recurrence, consider maintenance with fluconazole 100-200 mg (PO) weekly
Prognosis: Good response to therapy. Relapses are common

CMV Retinitis (Cytomegalovirus)

	Preferred Therapy	Alternate Therapy
Initial therapy	Initiate systemic CMV therapy* pending ophthalmology consult For immediate sight-threatening lesions Ganciclovir (GCV) intraocular implant plus valganciclovir 900 mg (PO) q12h for at least 21 days; can reduce dose to maintenance therapy (below) when retinitis deemed inactive by consulting ophthalmologist For peripheral lesions Valganciclovir 900 mg (PO) q12h x 21 days	Initiate systemic CMV therapy* pending ophthalmology consult Ganciclovir 5 mg/kg (IV) q12h x 2-3 weeks, then either 5 mg/kg (IV) q24h or valganciclovir 900 mg (PO) q24h **or** Foscarnet 60 mg/kg (IV) q8h or 90 mg/kg (IV) q12h x 3 weeks, then 90–120 mg/kg (IV) q24h **or** Cidofovir 5 mg/kg (IV) x 2 weeks, then every 2 weeks. Give probenecid 2 gm (PO) 3 hours before and 1 gm (PO) 2 and 8 hours after cidofovir (total of 4 gm)
Maintenance therapy	Valganciclovir 900 mg (PO) q24h indefinitely **or** Foscarnet 90–120 mg/kg (IV) q24h indefinitely	Cidofovir 5 mg/kg (IV) every other week with probenecid as above **or** Fomivirsen 1 vial (330 mg) injected into vitreous, then repeated every 2-4 weeks

* *Length of high-dose induction therapy depends on rate of response to treatment, typically 2-4 weeks*

Clinical Presentation: Blurred vision, scotomata, field cuts common. Often bilateral, even when initial symptoms are unilateral

Diagnostic Considerations: Diagnosis by characteristic hemorrhagic ("tomato soup and milk") retinitis on funduscopic exam. Consult ophthalmology in suspected cases

Pitfalls: May develop immune reconstitution vitreitis after starting antiretroviral therapy

Therapeutic Considerations: Oral valganciclovir is the preferred option for initial and maintenance therapy. Life-long maintenance therapy for CMV retinitis is required for CD4 counts < 100/mm^3, but may be discontinued if CD4 counts increase to > 100-150/mm^3 for 6 or more months in response to antiretroviral therapy (in consultation with ophthalmologist). Patients with CMV retinitis who discontinue therapy should undergo regular eye exams to monitor for relapse. Ganciclovir intraocular implants might need to be replaced every 6–8 months for patients who remain immunosuppressed with CD4 < 100-150/mm^3. Immune recovery uveitis (IRU) may develop in the setting of immune reconstitution due to ART and be treated by ophthalmologist with periocular corticosteroid ± systemic corticosteroid

Prognosis: Good initial response to therapy. High relapse rate unless CD4 improves with antiretroviral therapy

Coccidioidomycosis Infection *(C. immitis)*

Infection	Therapy*
Nonmeningeal infection	Acute therapy (diffuse pulmonary or disseminated disease) Amphotericin B deoxycholate 0.5-1.0 mg/kg (IV) q24h until clinical improvement (usually 500-1,000 mg total dose). Some specialists add an azole to amphotericin B therapy Acute therapy (milder disease) Fluconazole 400-800 mg (PO) q24h or Itraconazole 200 mg (PO) q12h Chronic maintenance therapy (secondary prophylaxis) Preferred: Fluconazole 400 mg (PO) q24h indefinitely; alternative: or Itraconazole 200 mg capsule (PO) q12h indefinitely
Meningeal infection*	Acute therapy Fluconazole 400-800 mg (IV) or (PO) q24h. Intrathecal amphotericin B if no response to azole therapy Chronic maintenance therapy (secondary prophylaxis) Fluconazole 400 mg (PO) q24h or itraconazole 200 mg capsule (PO) q12h indefinitely

* *Therapy for meningeal infection should be lifelong with fluconazole 400-800 mg q24h. There are insufficient data to recommend discontinuation of chronic maintenance therapy in other settings.*

Clinical Presentation: Typically a complication of advanced HIV infection (CD4 cell count < 200/mm^3). Most patients present with disseminated disease, which can manifest as fever, diffuse pulmonary infiltrates, adenopathy, skin lesions (multiple forms – verrucous, cold abscesses, ulcers, nodules), and/or bone lesions. Approximately 10% will have spread to the CNS in the form of meningitis (fever, headache, altered mental status)

Diagnostic Considerations: Consider the diagnosis in any patient with advanced HIV-related

immunosuppression who has been in a *C. immitis* endemic area (Southwestern US, northern Mexico) and presents with a systemic febrile syndrome. Diagnosis can be made by culture of the organism, visualization of characteristic spherules on histopathology, or a positive complement-fixation antibody (≥ 1:16). In meningeal cases, CSF profile shows low glucose, high protein, and lymphocytic pleocytosis
Pitfalls: Antibody titers are often negative on presentation. CSF profile of meningitis can be similar to TB
Prognosis: Related to extent of infection and degree of immunosuppression. Clinical response tends to be slow, especially with a high disease burden and advanced HIV disease. Meningeal disease is treated life-long regardless of CD4 recovery

Extrapulmonary Tuberculosis

Pathogen	Therapy
Mycobacterium tuberculosis	Treat the same as pulmonary TB (see p. 70). May require longer duration of therapy based on clinical response

Clinical Presentation: Multiple presentations possible (e.g., lymphadenitis, osteomyelitis, meningitis, hepatitis). Dissemination is more common in patients with low CD4 cell counts (< 100/mm^3)
Diagnostic Considerations: Diagnosis by isolator blood cultures or tissue biopsy
Pitfalls: Patients with disseminated disease frequently have pulmonary disease, which has implications for infection control
Therapeutic Considerations: Response to therapy may be slower than in normal hosts
Prognosis: Usually responsive to therapy

Herpes Simplex Virus (HSV) Disease

Infection	Preferred Therapy	Alternate Therapy
Orolabial lesions or initial/recurrent genital HSV	Famciclovir 500 mg (PO) q12h x 1-2 weeks **or** valacyclovir 1 gm (PO) q12h x 1-2 weeks **or** acyclovir 400 mg (PO) q8h x 1-2 weeks	Acyclovir-resistant HSV Foscarnet 60-100 mg/kg (IV) q12h until clinical response **or** Cidofovir 5 mg/kg (IV) weekly until clinical response
Moderate-to-severe mucocutaneous HSV	Initial therapy: Acyclovir 5 mg/kg (IV) q8h x 2-7 days. If improvement, switch to famciclovir 500 mg (PO) q12h **or** valacyclovir 1 gm (PO) q12h **or** acyclovir 400 mg (PO) q8h to complete 7-10 days	Acyclovir-resistant HSV Foscarnet 60-100 mg/kg (IV) q12h until clinical response **or** Cidofovir 5 mg/kg (IV) weekly until clinical response

Herpes Simplex Virus (HSV) Disease

Infection	Preferred Therapy	Alternate Therapy
HSV keratitis	Trifluridine 1% ophthalmic solution, one drop onto cornea q2h, not to exceed 9 drops per day and no longer than 21 days. Treatment in conjunction with ophthalmology consultation	Acyclovir-resistant HSV Foscarnet 60-100 mg/kg (IV) q12h until clinical response **or** Cidofovir 5 mg/kg (IV) weekly until clinical response
HSV encephalitis	Acyclovir 10 mg/kg (IV) q8h x 2-3 weeks	Acyclovir-resistant HSV Foscarnet 60-100 mg/kg (IV) q12h until clinical response **or** Cidofovir 5 mg/kg (IV) weekly until clinical response
Multiple mucocutaneous (oral or anogenital) relapses (chronic suppressive therapy)	Acyclovir 400 mg (PO) q12h **or** Famciclovir 250 mg (PO) q12h **or** Valacyclovir 500 mg (PO) q12h	Patients may be able to titrate dose downward to maintain response

Herpes Simplex (genital/oral)

Clinical Presentation: Painful, grouped vesicles on an erythematous base that rupture, crust, and heal within 2 weeks. Lesions may be chronic, severe, ulcerative with advanced immunosuppression

Diagnostic Considerations: Diagnosis by viral culture of swab from lesion base/roof of blister; alternative diagnostic techniques include Tzanck prep or immunofluorescence staining

Pitfalls: Acyclovir prophylaxis is not required in patients receiving ganciclovir or foscarnet

Therapeutic Considerations: In refractory cases, consider acyclovir resistance and treat with foscarnet. Topical trifluridine ophthalmic solution (Viroptic 1%) may be considered for direct application to small, localized areas of refractory disease; clean with hydrogen peroxide, then debride lightly with gauze, apply trifluridine, and cover with bacitracin/polymyxin ointment and nonadsorbent gauze; topical cidofovir (requires compounding) also may be tried. Chronic suppressive therapy with oral acyclovir, famciclovir, or valacyclovir may be indicated for patients with frequent recurrences, dosing similar to HIV-negative patients

Prognosis: Responds well to treatment except in severely immunocompromised patients, in whom acyclovir resistance may develop. Prognosis for HSV meningitis is excellent

Herpes Encephalitis (HSV-1)

Clinical Presentation: Acute onset of fever and change in mental status

Diagnostic Considerations: EEG is abnormal early (< 72 hours), showing unilateral temporal lobe abnormalities. Brain MRI is abnormal before CT scan, which may require several days before a temporal lobe focus is seen. Definitive diagnosis is by CSF PCR for HSV-1 DNA. Profound decrease in sensorium is characteristic of HSV meningoencephalitis. CSF may have PMN predominance and low glucose levels, unlike other viral causes of meningitis. A different clinical entity is HSV meningitis, which is usually associated with HSV-2 and can recur with

lymphocytic meningitis
Pitfalls: Rule out non-infectious causes of encephalopathy. Surprisingly, HSV encephalitis is a relatively rare cause of encephalitis in patients with HIV
Therapeutic Considerations: Treat as soon as possible since neurological deficits may be mild and reversible early on, but severe and irreversible later
Prognosis: Related to extent of brain injury and early antiviral therapy. Prognosis for HSV meningitis is excellent

Histoplasmosis *(H. capsulatum)*, Disseminated

Subset	Preferred Therapy	Alternate Therapy
Acute phase (3-10 days or until clinically improved)	Amphotericin B deoxycholate 0.7 mg/kg (IV) q24h or liposomal amphotericin B 4 mg/kg (IV) q24h*	Itraconazole 400 mg (IV) q24h*
Continuation phase	Itraconazole 200 mg capsule (PO) q12h x 12 weeks (consider q8h dosing on days 1-3)	Itraconazole oral solution 200 mg (PO) q12h x 12 weeks **or** Fluconazole 800 mg (PO) q24h x 12 weeks
Meningitis	Amphotericin B deoxycholate 0.7 mg/kg (IV) q24h x 12-16 weeks **or** Liposomal amphotericin B 4 mg/kg (IV) q24h x 12–16 weeks	Fluconazole 800 mg (PO) q24h x 12 weeks

* *Duration of therapy dependent on response to therapy*

Clinical Presentation: Two general forms: Mild disease with fever/lymph node enlargement (e.g., cervical adenitis), or severe disease with fever, wasting ± diarrhea/meningitis/GI ulcerations
Diagnostic Considerations: Diagnosis by urine/serum histoplasmosis antigen, sometimes by culture of bone marrow/liver or isolator blood cultures. May occur in patients months to years after having lived/moved from an endemic area
Pitfalls: Relapse is common after discontinuation of therapy. Cultures may take 7-21 days to turn positive. Itraconazole has many drug-drug interactions with antiretrovirals
Therapeutic Considerations: Initial therapy depends on severity of illness on presentation. Extremely sick patients should be started on amphotericin B deoxycholate, with duration of IV therapy dependent on response to treatment. Mildly ill patients can be started on itraconazole. All patients require chronic suppressive therapy, with possible discontinuation for immune reconstitution with CD4 counts > 100/mm^3 for at least 6 months. HIV patients with CD4 > 500/mm^3 and acute pulmonary histoplasmosis might not require therapy, but a short course of itraconazole (4-8 weeks) is reasonable to prevent systemic spread
Prognosis: Usually responds to treatment, except in fulminant cases

Human Papillomavirus (HPV) Disease

Infection	Patient-Applied Therapy	Provider-Applied Therapy
Condyloma acuminata (genital warts)	Podofilox 0.5% solution or 0.5% gel to all lesions q12h x 3 consecutive days, then repeat weekly for up to 4 weeks **or** Imiquimod 5% cream to all lesions at bedtime and remove in the morning on 3 non-consecutive nights weekly for up to 16 weeks	Liquid nitrogen cryotherapy to each lesion until thoroughly frozen, then repeat every 1-2 weeks for up to 3-4 times **or** Trichloroacetic acid or bichloracetic acid cauterization 80%-95% aqueous solution to all lesions, then repeat weekly for up to 3-6 weeks **or** Surgical excision or laser surgery **or** Podophyllin resin 10%-25% suspension in tincture of benzoin to all lesions and wash off in a few hours, then repeat weekly for up to 3-6 weeks
Cervical intraepithelial neoplasia (CIN)	<u>CIN 1</u>: Pap smears and/or colposcopy every 4-6 months <u>CIN 2 or 3</u>: Loop electrosurgical excision procedure (LEEP)	<u>CIN 2 or 3</u>: Cryotherapy or laser therapy or cone biopsy. Low-dose intravaginal 5-fluorouracil 2 gm twice weekly x 6 months may reduce short-term risk for recurrence
Anal intraepithelial neoplasia (AIN)	Insufficient data to recommend specific treatment; decision based on size, location of lesion, and grade of histology. Efficacy of treatment of AIN-2 or AIN-3 for prevention of anal cancer is unknown	

Genital/Perianal Warts (Condyloma Acuminata)

Clinical Presentation: Single/multiple verrucous genital lesions ± pigmentation usually without inguinal adenopathy

Diagnostic Considerations: Diagnosis by clinical appearance. Genital warts are usually caused by HPV types 11,16. Anogenital warts caused by HPV types 16,18,31,33,35 are associated with cervical neoplasia

Pitfalls: Most HPV infections are asymptomatic

Therapeutic Considerations: First-line therapy is ablative (cryotherapy or cauterization); if no response to standard treatment, attempt to treat with surgery or cidofovir. Intralesional interferon-alfa generally is not recommended

Prognosis: Related to HPV serotypes with malignant potential (HPV types 16,18,31,33,35). The rate of recurrence of anogenital warts is high despite treatment

Mycobacterium Avium Complex (MAC) Disease

Pathogen	Preferred Therapy	Alternate Therapy
Mycobacterium avium complex	At least 2 drugs as initial therapy Clarithromycin 500 mg (PO) q12h plus ethambutol 15 mg/kg (PO) q24h (usually 800 mg or 1200 mg daily). Consider adding third drug, rifabutin 300 mg (PO) q24h, for patients with CD4 < 50/mm^3, high mycobacterial loads and severely symptomatic disease. Duration of therapy is **lifelong**, although consider discontinuation in asymptomatic patients with > 12 months therapy and CD4 > 100/mm^3 for > 6 months in response to ART	Alternative to clarithromycin Azithromycin 500-600 mg (PO) q24h Alternative 3rd or 4th drug for severe symptoms or disseminated disease Ciprofloxacin 500-750 mg (PO) q12h **or** Levofloxacin 500 mg (PO) q24h **or** Amikacin 10-15 mg/kg (IV) q24h

Clinical Presentation: Typically presents as a febrile wasting illness in advanced HIV disease (CD4 < 50/mm^3). Focal invasive disease is possible, especially in patients with advanced immunosuppression after starting antiretroviral therapy. Focal disease likely reflects restoration of pathogen-specific immune response to subclinical infection ("immune reconstitution inflammatory syndrome" [IRIS]), and typically manifests as lymphadenitis (mesenteric, cervical, thoracic) or rarely disease in the spine mimicking Pott's disease. Immune reconstitution syndrome usually occurs within weeks to months after starting antiretroviral therapy for the first time, but may occur a year or more later

Diagnostic Considerations: Diagnosis by isolation of organism from a normally sterile body site (blood, lymph node, bone marrow, liver biopsy). Lysis centrifugation (DuPont isolator) is the preferred blood culture method. Anemia/↑ alkaline phosphatase are occasionally seen

Pitfalls: Isolator blood cultures may be negative, especially in immune reconstitution inflammatory syndrome initially

Therapeutic Considerations: Some studies suggest benefit for addition of rifabutin 300 mg (PO) q24h, others do not. Rifabutin may require dosage adjustment with NNRTI's and PI's (see p. 70). For concurrent use with nelfinavir, indinavir, or amprenavir, decrease rifabutin to 150 mg (PO) q24h. For concurrent use with ritonavir, decrease rifabutin to 150 mg (PO) 2-3x/week. For concurrent use with efavirenz, increase rifabutin to 450-600 mg (PO) q24h. The dose of PI's or NNRTI's may need to be increased by 20-25%. Monitor carefully for rifabutin drug toxicity (arthralgias, uveitis, leukopenia). Treat IRIS initially with NSAIDs; if symptoms persist, systemic corticosteroids (prednisone 20-40 mg daily) for 4-8 weeks can be used. Some patients will require a more prolonged course of corticosteroids with a slow taper over months. Azithromycin is often better tolerated than clarithromycin and has fewer drug-drug interactions. Optimal long-term management is unknown, though most studies suggest that treatment can be discontinued in asymptomatic patients with > 12 months of therapy and CD4 > 100/mm^3 for > 6 months

Prognosis: Depends on immune reconstitution in response to antiretroviral therapy. Adverse prognostic factors include high-grade bacteremia or severe wasting

Syphilis *(Treponema pallidum)*

Stage	Preferred Therapy	Alternate Therapy
Early (primary, secondary, early latent)	Benzathine penicillin G 2.4 million U (IM) x 1 dose	Doxycycline 100 mg (PO) q12h x 14 days **or** Ceftriaxone 1 gm (IV) q24h x 10 days
Late latent (≥1 year or unknown duration, no CNS involvement)	Benzathine penicillin G 2.4 million U (IM) weekly x 3 weeks	Doxycycline 100 mg (PO) q12h x 28 days
Late (aortitis and gummata)	Infectious diseases consultation	Infectious diseases consultation
Neurosyphilis (includes otic and ocular disease)	Aqueous crystalline penicillin G 2–4 million U (IV) q4h (or total dose by continuous IV infusion) x 14 days **followed by** Benzathine penicillin G 2.4 million U (IM) weekly x 3 weeks after completion of (IV) therapy	Procaine penicillin 2.4 MU (IM) q24h x 14 days plus probenecid 500 mg (PO) q6h x 14 days (cannot use if sulfonamide-allergic) **with or without** Benzathine penicillin G 2.4 MU (IM) weekly x 3 weeks after completion of above For penicillin-allergic patients Ceftriaxone 2 gm (IV) q24h x 14 days

Epidemiology: Syphilis is highly prevalent among some groups with high rates of HIV, notably gay men. Studies have shown that syphilis facilitates HIV transmission, and case reports/series suggest that syphilis in HIV-infected patients is associated with multiple and slower resolving primary chancres, higher titer RPR, slower decline of RPR titers, higher rate of serologic failure, increased frequency of CSF abnormalities and CSF-VDRL positivity, higher incidence of ocular disease, and higher rates of relapse after treatment (Sex Transm Dis 2001 28:158-65; N Engl J Med 1997 Jul 337:307-14; Ann Intern Med 1990; 113:872)

Clinical Presentation: The causative organism of syphilis is *Treponema pallidum*, which cannot be cultured in routine clinical laboratories. As a result, the diagnosis of syphilis depends on recognizing the clinical stages and use of serologic tests

- Primary syphilis: Following an incubation period of 2-6 weeks, primary syphilis presents as a papule that later ulcerates to form a syphilitic chancre. These are generally painless and may occur on any mucosal surface. Non-tender regional adenopathy may also be present. Serologic tests for syphilis (RPR or VDRL) can be negative early in primary syphilis, so empiric treatment is indicated in suspected cases, with follow-up testing necessary to confirm the disease
- Secondary syphilis: Approximately 60-90% of patients with untreated primary syphilis will develop secondary syphilis as a manifestation of *T. pallidum* dissemination. The time course is typically within 6 months of infection acquisition, and the clinical manifestations

are highly variable. The most common manifestation of secondary syphilis is a non-pruritic macular-papular rash over the entire body, including the palms and soles. Other symptoms and laboratory abnormalities can include condyloma lata (white genital lesions similar in appearance to condyloma acuminata), mucous patches (shallow ulcerations on the oral or genital mucosa), fever, malaise, lymphadenopathy, anorexia, hepatitis, and diminished vision secondary to uveitis

- Latent syphilis: Defined by a reactive serologic test in the absence of active symptoms, latent syphilis is divided into "early-latent" (< 1 year after exposure) and "late-latent" (> 1 year after exposure). Patients who are unable to give an accurate exposure date are classified as "latent syphilis of unknown duration" and treated as late-latent disease
- Tertiary (late) syphilis: This develops in 25-40% of patients untreated for earlier disease, usually months to years later. Tertiary syphilis can cause CNS disease, cardiovascular disorders, and gummatous lesions involving the skin and bones. Cardiovascular and gummatous syphilis have become extremely rare, but CNS syphilis still occurs with some frequency and can present in various ways. *Acute syphilitic meningitis* and *meningovascular syphilis* occur relatively early after exposure (typically within the first 1-5 years), sometimes during dissemination of the organism with secondary syphilis. By contrast, *parenchymatous syphilis* usually occurs decades later, and includes general paresis, tabes dorsalis, and focal lesions due to CNS gummas

Diagnostic Considerations: Diagnostic strategies for syphilis are the same as in HIV-negative patients, and rely mostly on serologic studies since the organism cannot be cultured. Darkfield microscopy on fluid obtained from chancres or condyloma lata may demonstrate the characteristic spiral-shaped organism; however, this technique is of limited utility since it cannot be used in the absence of obvious lesions, and most clinicians do not have access to a darkfield microscope. As a result, a positive serologic test for syphilis (RPR or VDRL) followed by a positive confirmatory test (MHA-TP, FTA-ABS, or TP-PA) is the most common way to diagnose syphilis in patients with (or without) HIV. Although case reports have cited unusually high titers, false negative results, and delayed onset of seropositivity in patients with HIV infection, no alternative testing strategy is routinely recommended. Neurosyphilis is diagnosed via clinical presentation and CSF examination. In symptomatic neurosyphilis, presenting complaints may include cognitive dysfunction, motor or sensory deficits, cranial nerve palsies, ophthalmic or auditory symptoms, and symptoms or signs of meningitis. Diagnostic criteria for neurosyphilis by CSF examination vary, but one commonly used definition is a CSF white blood cell count > 20 cells/mcL or a reactive CSF VDRL. (Although considered highly sensitive, the FTA-ABS test of the spinal fluid is not specific and can be used only to rule out disease.) The diagnosis of neurosyphilis is challenging since the CSF VDRL (the most specific test) is positive in only 30-70%, even in HIV negative-patients. Furthermore, HIV itself may induce cellular responses independent of syphilis, and clinical manifestations are extremely varied. As a result, there is some debate about which patients with HIV and syphilis should undergo lumbar puncture (LP). One study of 326 HIV infected patients with syphilis who underwent LP found that 65 (20%) met criteria for neurosyphilis by CSF exam; the risk was substantially higher if the CD4 cell count was ≤ 350 or the RPR was ≥ 1:32 (J Infect Dis 2004;189:369-76). Based on this study, the diagnostic approach shown in Table 5.3 is reasonable

Therapeutic Considerations: The treatment of syphilis is generally the same as for HIV-negative patients, with penicillin as the mainstay of therapy. The criteria for treatment response are the same in HIV-infected and HIV-negative individuals. Specifically, the RPR or VDRL titer should decline ≥ 4–fold by one year after treatment for early syphilis and by 2-3 years after treatment for latent syphilis. (For HIV patients with early syphilis, there is an increased rate of treatment failure when using serologic criteria; therefore, our practice is to include an RPR as part of monitoring labs performed every 3-4 months unless the titer has reverted to negative.) Failure to achieve ≥ 4–fold decline in titer should prompt investigation of reinfection or a CSF examination to exclude neurosyphilis. For patients with neurosyphilis, follow-up CSF examinations are performed every 6 months until CSF pleocytosis has normalized; if still abnormal 2 years after treatment, consider retreatment with intravenous penicillin

Table 5.3. Need for Lumbar Puncture (LP) in HIV-Infected Patients with Syphilis

Stage of Syphilis	RPR	CD4	Recommendation
Primary, secondary, or early latent	Any	Any	No LP; if RPR > 1:32 or CD4 < 350, be especially vigilant for lack of response
Late-latent or syphilis of unknown duration	< 1:32	> 350	No LP (some experts recommend LP for all HIV patients with latent syphilis)
	> 1:32	Any	Perform LP
	Any	< 350	Perform LP
Positive RPR and confirmatory test with neurologic, ophthalmic, or auditory symptoms/signs	Any	Any	Perform LP

Varicella Zoster Virus (VZV) Disease

Infection	Preferred Therapy
Primary VZV infection (chickenpox)	Acyclovir 10 mg/kg (IV) q8h x 7–10 days. Can start with or change to oral therapy with valacyclovir 1 gm (PO) q8h or famciclovir 500 mg (PO) q8h after defervescence if no evidence of visceral involvement exists
Local dermatomal herpes zoster	Famciclovir 500 mg (PO) q8h x 7-10 days **or** Valacyclovir 1 gm (PO) q8h x 7–10 days
Extensive cutaneous lesion or visceral involvement	Acyclovir 10 mg/kg (IV) q8h until cutaneous and visceral disease has clearly resolved and the patient is clinically improved
Acute retinal necrosis	Acyclovir 10 mg/kg (IV) q8h until progression stops, then valacyclovir 1 gm (PO) q8h x 6 weeks. Treat in conjunction with close ophthalmologic consultation

Clinical Presentation: Primary varicella (chickenpox) presents as clear vesicles on an erythematous base that heal with crusting and sometimes scarring. Zoster usually presents as painful tense vesicles on an erythematous base in a dermatomal distribution. In patients with HIV, primary varicella is more severe/prolonged, and zoster is more likely to involve multiple dermatomes/disseminate. VZV can rarely cause acute retinal necrosis, which requires close consultation with ophthalmology

Diagnostic Considerations: Diagnosis is usually clinical. In atypical cases, immunofluorescence can be used to distinguish herpes zoster from herpes simplex

Pitfalls: Extend treatment beyond 7-10 days if new vesicles are still forming after initial treatment period. Corticosteroids for dermatomal zoster are not recommended in HIV-positive patients

Therapeutic Considerations: IV therapy is generally indicated for severe disease/cranial nerve zoster

Prognosis: Usually responds slowly to treatment

Hepatitis Coinfection

Hepatitis C Infection

Pathogen	Therapy
Hepatitis C virus (HCV)	Peginterferon alfa-2b 1.5 mcg/kg (SQ) weekly* or Peginterferon alfa-2a 180 mcg (SQ) weekly* **plus** Ribavirin† (PO) (weight-based dosing: if < 75 mg, 400 mg in morning and 600 mg in evening; if > 75 kg, 600 mg q12h)

* *Duration of therapy (all genotypes): 48 weeks for patients who demonstrate an early virologic response (> 2 log decrease in HCV viral load at 12 weeks); 12 weeks for patients who fail to achieve an early virologic response at 12 weeks (therapy beyond 12 weeks is almost always futile for achieving virologic cure)*

† *Monotherapy (peginterferon alfa-2b or alfa-2a) is indicated in patients with a contraindication to ribavirin (e.g., unstable cardiopulmonary disease, pre-existing anemia, hemoglobinopathy)*

Epidemiology: Hepatitis C virus (HCV) infection is transmitted primarily through blood exposure; sexual and perinatal transmission are also possible but less efficient. A notable exception is sexually transmitted HCV among gay men. Since modes of transmission of HIV and HCV are similar, there are high rates of HCV coinfection in HIV – an estimated 16% of HIV patients overall, including 80% or more of IDUs and 5-10% of gay men (Clin Infect Dis 2002;34:831-7). Genotype 1 accounts for 75% of HCV in the US. HIV accelerates the progression of chronic HCV infection to cirrhosis, liver failure, and hepatocellular carcinoma (J Infect Dis 2001;183:1112-5; Clin Infect Dis 2001;33:562-569). Data are conflicting regarding the independent effect of HCV on HIV disease progression, but several studies have shown a markedly higher rate of antiretroviral therapy-induced hepatotoxicity in those with chronic HCV. In some series, liver failure from HCV is one of the leading causes of death in HIV/HCV coinfected individuals (Clin Infect Dis 2001;32:492-7)

Clinical Presentation: Persistently elevated liver transaminases; usually asymptomatic

Diagnostic Considerations: All HIV-positive patients should be tested for HCV antibody. If the antibody test is negative but the likelihood of HCV infection is high (IDU, unexplained increase in LFTs), obtain an HCV RNA since false-negative antibody tests may occur, especially in advanced HIV disease (J Clin Microbiol 2000;38:575-7). Since LFT elevation does not correlate well with underlying HCV activity, a liver biopsy is the best way to assess the degree of fibrosis and inflammation

Therapeutic Considerations:

Once Diagnosis is Established. Advise patients to abstain from alcohol and administer vaccinations for hepatitis A and B (if non-immune). Also obtain HCV RNA levels with genotype assessment. HCV RNA levels do not have prognostic significance for underlying degree of liver disease, but higher levels make treatment for cure less likely. Genotype results also correlate with cure rates (reported cure rates: 60-75% for genotypes 2 and 3; 15-25% for genotype 1). Some clinicians elect to treat HCV without a liver biopsy due to: the risks, costs, and discomfort of the test; the potential to underestimate the degree of HCV activity due to sampling error; and the high rate of treatment success for genotypes 2 and 3

Optimal Patient Characteristics for HCV Treatment in HIV include no active psychiatric disease or substance abuse; stable HIV disease with undetectable HIV RNA and higher CD4 cell count; receiving an antiretroviral regimen that does not contain ddI (in particular), d4T, or ZDV; and adherent to medications, follow-up visits, and blood test monitoring. Only a small proportion of patients will meet all these criteria; therefore, to maximize treatment effect, it is important to optimize clinical status prior to starting HCV therapy. Patients should be fully educated regarding the goals and risks of treatment, with provision of written information about side effects, local support groups, and whom to contact with questions. It is useful to administer the first dose of treatment in the office in order to provide instructions on injection techniques

Choice of Drug Therapy. The treatment of choice for HCV infection is pegylated interferon plus ribavirin. All patients should also receive hepatitis A vaccine and counseling to avoid alcohol use

- Pegylated Interferon. Two different formulations of pegylated interferon are available for treatment of HCV infection: (1) peginterferon alfa-2a (Pegasys), supplied as a pre-mixed solution and administered subcutaneously as a fixed dose of 180 mcg once a week; and (2) peginterferon alfa-2b (Peg-Intron), supplied as a powder that is reconstituted in saline and administered subcutaneously as a weight-based dose once a week. Efficacy and toxicity of these two peginterferon preparations appear to be similar. Three clinical trials have shown that pegylated interferon plus ribavirin is more effective than standard interferon plus ribavirin (N Engl J Med 2004;351:451-9; N Engl J Med 2004;351:438-50; JAMA 2004;292:2839-48). Interferon has numerous side effects, the most important of which are listed in Table 5.4.
- Ribavirin. Ribavirin is available in 200–mg capsules. Although the dose used in clinical trials was 800 mg daily (400 mg bid), it appears that a higher initial dose is associated with greater efficacy. Standard dose is now 400 mg qAM and 600 mg qPM for weight < 75 kg, and 600 mg qAM and 600 mg qPM for weight > 75 kg. Ribavirin causes hemolytic anemia that predictably leads to a measurable decline in hemoglobin; this stabilizes by week 4-8 of treatment. Hemolytic anemia may be exacerbated in patients receiving ZDV; if possible an alternative NRTI should be chosen, with preference for tenofovir or abacavir. For symptomatic anemia or patients with coexisting conditions exacerbated by anemia, erythropoietin is used to maintain hemoglobin levels > 10 gm/dL or higher as needed. The typical starting dose of erythropoietin is 40,000 units SQ once a week. ddI is contraindicated during ribavirin administration due to an increased risk of mitochondrial toxicity and hepatic decompensation (Clin Infect Dis 2004;38:e79-e80). d4T should also be avoided because of its potential for inducing mitochondrial toxicity itself. Finally, some data suggest that ABC may interact with ribavirin, reducing efficacy of HCV therapy.

Another common side effect of ribavirin is GI distress, which can overlap with a similar effect of interferon. Ribavirin is pregnancy category X (potent teratogen), and can only be used in sexually-active women of childbearing potential if they are using 2 forms of birth control. Pregnancy should be avoided until at least 6 months after stopping ribavirin.

Monitoring. The monitoring plan for HIV/HCV coinfected patients consists of both safety and efficacy evaluations (Table 5.5). Results of HCV RNA testing are used to decide between completing 48 weeks of HCV therapy vs. discontinuing treatment at 12 or 24 weeks due to low probability of cure (Figure 5.1)

Table 5.4. Adverse Effects Associated with Interferon

Side Effect	Comments
Fatigue and flu-like symptoms (fever, chills, muscle aches, headache)	Dose at night so that some initial symptoms can be slept through. Symptoms may not peak until 48-78 hours after weekly dose and can be managed with acetaminophen (maximum 1300 mg/day) or ibuprofen plus good hydration. Fatigue is sometimes a manifestation of thyroid dysregulation or anemia; monitor thyroid function tests and CBC
Depression	Interferon can aggravate life-threatening psychiatric conditions. Low threshold for initiating anti-depressant therapy. Patients with a pre-existing history of depression or other psychiatric disease should be followed closely by mental health professionals during HCV treatment
Leukopenia, thrombocytopenia, anemia	Cytopenias are more common in HIV/HCV co-infection. Can treat with G-CSF 300 mcg 3x/week if absolute neutrophil count is < 500/mm^3. If neutropenia persists, decrease dose of interferon. If platelet count falls to < 80,000/mm^3, also consider decreasing interferon dose (some clinicians tolerate counts down to 50,000/mm^3. Low threshold for use of erythropoietin (EPO) 40,000 U/week for anemia (see section on ribavirin)
Mouth ulcers	Topical viscous lidocaine or sucralfate is helpful in some
Gastrointestinal symptoms	Nausea and anorexia are the most common, often leading to weight loss. Advise patients to eat several small meals daily rather than a few large meals
Hair loss	Reversible after completion of therapy

Table 5.5. Monitoring Plan During Treatment for HCV infection

	Weeks of Treatment								
	Baseline	**2**	**4**	**8**	**12**	**16**	**20**	**24**	**24-48**
CBC	X	X	X	X	X	X	X	X	q4 weeks
LFTs + metabolic panel	X		X	X	X	X	X	X	q4 weeks
HCV RNA	X		±¶		X*			X**	q12 weeks
HIV RNA + CD4 profile	X				X†			X	q12 weeks
TSH	X				X			X	q12 weeks
Depression	X	X	X	X	X	X	X	X	ongoing
Ophthalmologic exam	X‡				X			X	q12 weeks
PT	X				X				q12 weeks
Pregnancy test	Perform at regular intervals if appropriate								

* Patients who have not dropped ≥ 2 logs from baseline HCV RNA at 12 weeks have < 3% chance of obtaining a sustained viral response (undetectable HCV RNA 6 months post-treatment). Discontinuation of therapy should be based on goal of treatment (i.e., viral eradication vs. histologic improvement).

** If undetectable HCV RNA at 24 weeks, continue therapy for an additional 24 weeks (if known genotype 2 or 3 discuss option to stop, but some experts agree co-infected patients should continue treatment for 48 weeks to decrease risk of relapse). If HCV RNA is positive at 24 weeks, consider discontinuing HCV therapy. Even in patients without viral response, treatment may improve liver histology. Also see Figure 5.1.

† *Anticipate decrease in absolute cell count but stable CD4%.*

‡ Necessary for patients with a history of retinopathy; IFN package insert recommends screening for all patients prior to treatment. Many clinicians choose to defer the initial exam and monitor for disturbances in vision and loss of color perception.

¶ Some check HCV RNA at week 4; if no decline in HIV RNA is seen, response is unlikely. In contrast, ≥ 1 log decline can be very motivating and treatment should be continued.

Adapted from: Brown, et al. Clinician's Guide to HIV/HCV Coinfection, June, 2004.

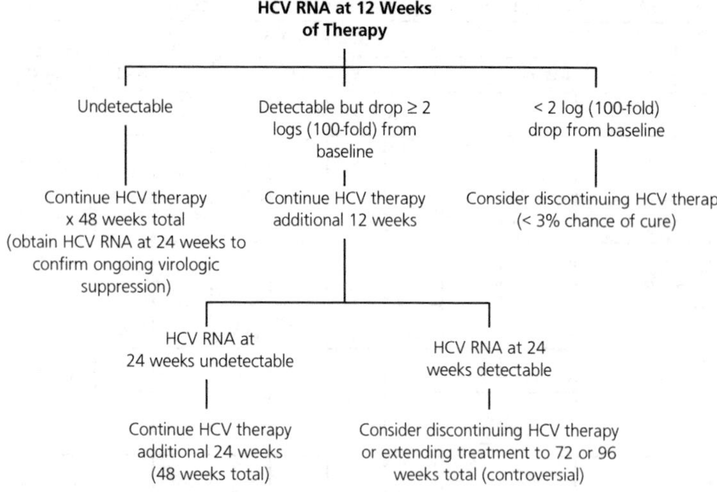

Figure 5.1. Management of HCV Infection Based on HCV RNA Testing

HCV RNA should be assessed at week 12. If the HCV viral load has not dropped by more than 2 logs (100-fold), then the likelihood of achieving a cure is extremely low. Many patients and providers will elect to discontinue therapy at this point. HCV RNA should be measured at weeks 24 and 48. If undetectable at week 48, additional measurements should be obtained at weeks 4, 12, and 24 after stopping treatment. An undetectable HCV RNA at week 24 post-treatment is the current standard for assessing a "sustained virologic response" (SVR), which can be equated with cure. Importantly, patients cured of HCV are susceptible to re-acquisition and should be cautioned about resuming high-risk behavior.

Internet Resources:

- HIV/HCV Co-infection Center of Excellence: www.uchsc.edu/mpaetc/coinfection
- AIDSinfo: www.aidsinfo.nih.gov
- Chronic Hepatitis C: Current Disease Management: www.niddk.nig.gov/
- Hep C Connection: www.hepc-connection.org
- Hepatitis Resource Network (HRN): www.h-r-n.org
- HIV and Hepatitis.com: www.hivandhepatitis.com
- Johns Hopkins Hepatitis C and HIV Coinfection Information: www.hopkins-hepc.org
- Management of Hepatitis C: 2002, NIH Consensus Statement: http://consensus.nih.gov/cons/cons.htm
- National HIV/AIDS Clinicians' Consultation Center: www.ucsf.ed/hivcntr
- The National AIDS Treatment Advocacy Project: www.natap.org
- Projects in Knowledge: www.projectsinknowledge.com

Hepatitis B Infection

HBV/HIV Status		
Need to Treat HIV	**Need to Treat HBV**	**Recommendation***
Yes	No	TDF plus either 3TC or FTC is the preferred NRTI backbone. Avoid monotherapy with TDF, 3TC, or FTC to reduce the risk of selecting HBV resistance
Yes	Yes	TDF plus either 3TC or FTC is the preferred NRTI backbone. Avoid monotherapy with TDF, 3TC, or FTC to reduce the risk of selecting HBV resistance. If TDF cannot be used (e.g., underlying renal disease), add entecavir to reduce the risk of selecting for 3TC or FTC resistance
No	Yes	In general, patients who need HBV treatment should also receive fully suppressive anti-HIV regimens, with the NRTI combination of choice being TDF plus either FTC or 3TC. However, in rare circumstances when HIV treatment is not an option or desired, pegylated interferon-alpha may be used as it does not select for HIV drug resistance. Another less desirable option is adefovir at a dose of 10 mg daily; while adefovir has HBV activity but not HIV activity at this dose, there is still the theoretical possibility of selecting for HIV drug resistance since higher doses of adefovir do have anti-HIV activity.
Need to discontinue NRTI's (TDF, 3TC, or FTC) with anti-HBV activity		Monitor clinical course with frequent liver function tests and consider the use of interferon, adefovir (10 mg daily), or telbivudine to prevent flares, especially in patients with marginal hepatic reserve

* *TDF, 3TC, and FTC should be administered at standard doses used for HIV infection (TDF 300 mg qd, 3TC 300 mg qd, FTC 200 mg qd)*

Epidemiology: Hepatitis B virus (HBV) infection is relatively common in patients with HIV, with approximately 60% showing some evidence of prior exposure. Chronic hepatitis B infection interacts with HIV infection in several important ways:

- HBV increases the risk of liver-related death and hepatotoxicity from antiretroviral therapy (Lancet 2002; 360:1921-6; Hepatology 2002;35:182-9)
- 3TC, FTC, and tenofovir each have anti-HBV activity. Thus selection of antiretroviral therapy for patients with HBV can have clinical and resistance implications for HBV as well as HIV. This is most notable with 3TC and FTC, as a high proportion of coinfected patients will develop HBV-associated resistance to these drugs after several years of therapy. This resistance reduces response to subsequent non-3TC or FTC anti-HBV therapy
- Cessation of anti-HBV therapy may lead to exacerbations of underlying liver disease; in some cases, these flares have been fatal (Clin Infect Dis 1999;28:1032-5; Scand J Infectious Diseases 2004;36:533-5)

- Immune reconstitution may lead to worsening of liver status, presumably because HBV disease is immune mediated. This is sometimes associated with loss of HBEAg
- Entecavir can no longer be recommended for HIV/HBV coinfected patients, as it has anti-HIV activity and may select for HIV resistance mutation M184V (N Engl J Med 2007;356:2614-21). If needed, it should be used only with a fully suppressive HIV regimen

Diagnostic Consideration: Obtain HBSAb, HBSAg, and HBCAb at baseline in all patients. If negative, hepatitis B vaccination is indicated. If chronic HBV infection (positive HBSAg) is identified, obtain HBEAg, HBEAb, and HBV DNA levels. As with HCV infection, vaccination with hepatitis A vaccine and counseling to avoid alcohol are important components of preventive care. Isolated Hepatitis B Core Antibody: Many patients with HIV have antibody to hepatitis B core (anti-HBc) but are negative for both HBSAg and HBSAb. This phenomenon appears to be more common in those with HCV coinfection (Clin Infec Dis 2003 36:1602-6). In this scenario, diagnostic considerations include: (1) recently acquired HBV, before development of HBSAb; (2) chronic HBV, with HBSAg below the levels of detection; (3) immunity to HBV, with HBSAb below the levels of detection; (4) false-positive anti-HBV core. As the incidence of HBV is relatively low in most populations and anti-HBc alone is usually a stable phenomenon over years, recent acquisition of HBV is rarely the explanation. We recommend checking HBV DNA in this situation: If positive, this indicates chronic HBV; if negative, then low-level immunity or false-positive anti-HBV core remain as possible explanations. It is useful to measure HBV serologic markers periodically in this population, as improvement in immune status due to ART may lead to increasing titers of HBSAb and subsequently confirm immunity (Clin Infect Dis 2007; 45:1221-9). In general, we do not recommend HBV immunization with isolated anti-HBc

Therapeutic Considerations: The optimal treatment for HBV infection is in evolution. Current guidelines suggest treatment of HBV in all patients with active HBV replication, defined as a detectable HBEAg or HBV DNA. Pending long-term studies defining optimal management, the recommendations set forth in the grid above are reasonable. Patients being treated with regimens for HBV should be monitored for ALT every 3-4 months. HBV DNA levels provide a good marker for efficacy of therapy and should be added to regular laboratory monitoring. The goal of therapy is to reduce HBV DNA to as low a level as possible, preferably below the limits of detection. The duration of HBV therapy is not well established; with development of HBEAb, while some individuals without HIV can stop therapy after reversion of HBEAg to negative, there are no clear stopping rules for HIV-coinfected patients

Opportunistic Infections Predominantly Outside USA/Canada/Europe

Paracoccidioidomycosis Infection

Pathogen	Preferred Therapy	Alternate Therapy
Paracoccidioides brasiliensis	Amphotericin B 0.5-1.0 mg/kg (IV) q24h for severely ill patients. Itraconazole 100–200 mg (PO) q24h for less ill patients	Ketoconazole 200–400 mg (PO) q24h **or** TMP-SMX 1 DS (PO) q12h

Pulmonary Paracoccidioidomycosis (South American Blastomycosis)

Clinical Presentation: Typically presents as a chronic pneumonia syndrome with productive cough, blood-tinged sputum, dyspnea, and chest pain. May also develop fever, malaise, weight loss, mucosal ulcerations in/around mouth and nose, dysphagia, changes in voice, cutaneous lesions on face/limbs, or cervical adenopathy. Can disseminate to prostate, epididymis, kidneys, or adrenals

Diagnostic Considerations: Characteristic "pilot wheel" shaped yeast in sputum. Diagnosis by culture and stain (Gomori) of organism from clinical specimen. Found only in Latin American. One-third of cases have only pulmonary involvement. Skin test is non-specific/non-diagnostic

Pitfalls: No distinguishing radiologic features. No clinical adrenal insufficiency, in contrast to TB or histoplasmosis. Hilar adenopathy/pleural effusions are uncommon

Therapeutic Considerations: Potent ART should be initiated in accordance with standards of care in the community. Chronic suppressive therapy with TMP-SMX 1 DS (PO) q24h should be continued indefinitely; no data on discontinuation of chronic maintenance therapy

Prognosis: Related to severity/extent of infection. HIV/AIDS require life-long suppression with TMP-SMX 1 DS tablet (PO) q24h or itraconazole 200 mg (PO) solution q24h

Penicillium Infection

Pathogen	Therapy
Penicillium marneffei	Acute infection in severely ill patients Amphotericin B 0.6 mg/kg /day (IV) x 2 weeks, then Itraconazole oral solution 400 mg (PO) q24h x 10 weeks Chronic maintenance therapy (secondary prophylaxis) Itraconazole 200 mg (PO) q24h

Cutaneous Penicillium (Penicillium marneffei)

Clinical Presentation: Papules, pustules, nodules, ulcers, or abscesses. Mostly seen in advanced HIV/AIDS

Diagnostic Considerations: Diagnosis by demonstrating organism by stain/culture in tissue specimen. Affects residents/visitors of Southeast Asia or Southern China

Pitfalls: Lesions commonly become umbilicated and resemble molluscum contagiosum

Therapeutic Considerations: ART should be administered according to standard of care in the community. Requires life-long suppressive therapy with itraconazole

Prognosis: Poor/fair. Related to degree of immunosuppression

Chapter 6
Complications of HIV Infection*

* Also see Chapter 5 for Opportunistic Infections and Chapters 3 and 9 for Drug-Induced Adverse Effects

HEMATOLOGIC COMPLICATIONS

A. Thrombocytopenia. May be the first and only sign of HIV infection. Treatment is only required for platelet count < 20,000/mm^3, active bleeding, or planned procedures. Causes include medications, alcohol, idiopathic thrombocytopenic purpura (ITP), thrombotic thrombocytopenic purpura (TTP), and advanced HIV disease ± marrow infiltration with secondary opportunistic infections (usually accompanied by pancytopenia)

1. **Idiopathic Thrombocytopenic Purpura (ITP).** Can occur at any stage of HIV disease and sometimes emerges as antiretroviral therapy induces an immune response. Consultation with a hematologist is advised for platelet count < 20,000 or if rapid recovery of platelet count is required.
   a. **Preferred therapy.** Combination antiretroviral therapy that includes ZDV (best studied agent for ITP). If ZDV-intolerant, ITP may still resolve with alternative combination regimens.
   b. **If rapid control of platelet count is needed.** IVIG 1-2 gm/kg total dose, over 2-5 days. Duration of response is typically 3-4 weeks. <u>Alternative</u>: Anti-RH D globulin (WinRho) 50-75 mcg/kg IV (effective only in RH-positive, non-splenectomized patients). Causes mild hemolysis. Duration of response is similar to IVIG, and may work in some patients who do not respond to IVIG
   c. **Miscellaneous alternative therapies.** Prednisone 1 mg/kg daily, with taper as tolerated; danazol 400-800 mg (PO) q24h; dapsone 100 mg (PO) q24h (if not G6PD-deficient); alpha-interferon 3 million units 3x/week; splenectomy. Some anecdotal evidence for use of vincristine, splenic irradiation, anti-cd20 antibody (Rituximab).
2. **Thrombotic Thrombocytopenic Purpura (TTP).** Manifests as microangiopathic hemolytic anemia associated with renal insufficiency and neurologic symptoms. TTP is a **medical emergency** – if is suspected based on clinical grounds and examination of blood smear, consult hematologist immediately. Standard treatment is prednisone 60-100 mg (PO) q24h (or IV equivalent) plus plasmapheresis.

B. Anemia. Anemia is associated with a lower quality of life and reduced survival (Clin Infect Dis 1999;29:44-9).

1. **Etiology**
   a. **Decreased RBC production (low reticulocyte count)**
      - **Direct effect of HIV** (usually CD4 < 100/mm^3); responds well to initiation of antiretroviral therapy
      - **Infiltration of bone marrow:** in particular MAC – suspect in a patient with advanced AIDS who has fever, weight loss, and anemia out of proportion to drop in other cell lines; can also be due to

lymphoma

- **Iron deficiency (women)**
- **B12 or folate deficiency:** a high MCV is usually related to a side effect of NRTI's (especially ZDV), but need to rule out B12 and folate deficiency, which appears to be more common among patients with HIV
- **Certain infections:** Parvovirus B19: infects and inhibits early RBC precursors, with characteristic bone marrow showing giant pronormoblasts; diagnosed by viral DNA by PCR of blood (not by serology); treated with IVIG. MAC: diagnosed by isolator blood cultures or bone marrow biopsy; treated as described on p. 88.
- **Drugs:** ZDV (most common in advanced HIV disease, but can occur at any stage; other antiretroviral agents rarely cause anemia); ganciclovir and valganciclovir (lower WBC also); TMP-SMX; amphotericin.

b. **Increased RBC destruction (high reticulocyte count)**
- **Drug-induced:** Dapsone and primaquine if patient is G6PD deficient; ribavirin as part of HCV therapy (causes dose-related hemolytic anemia), which may further compromise fatigue associated with HCV therapy.
- **TTP (described on p. 101)**

2. **Evaluation.** As a minimum work-up, evaluate clinical status, stage of HIV disease, stool for occult blood, CBC/differential, RBC indices, reticulocyte count, iron, TIBC, creatinine, LFTs, B12, folate. Bone marrow aspiration is indicated when above work-up and history fail to identify a cause.
3. **Treatment.** If no reversible cause of anemia is identified, or if the cause cannot be removed (for example, ribavirin-associated anemia during HCV treatment), consider erythropoietin (EPO) for patients with Hgb < 10 gm/dL or HCT < 30. Start with 40,000 units (SQ) once weekly with iron supplementation; if at 4 weeks, Hgb has increased by > 1 gm/dL, continue same dose until Hgb reaches 13 gm/dL. Dose can then be reduced to 10,000 units (SQ) once weekly to maintain Hgb at this level. Stop therapy for Hgb > 15 gm/dL. For non-responders, 60,000 units (SQ) once weekly may be effective.

C. **Neutropenia.** As with anemia, neutropenia is much more common in advanced HIV disease. The risk of infection is increased with lower absolute neutrophil counts (ANC), especially when < 500/mm^3.

1. **Etiology**

a. **Direct effect of HIV.** Responds well to initiation of antiretroviral therapy

b. **Drugs.** ZDV, ganciclovir and valganciclovir (ZDV and ganciclovir given together can cause particularly severe neutropenia), pyrimethamine, interferon (pegylated interferon more likely to cause neutropenia than standard interferon), flucytosine. Uncommon causes include other NRTI's, ribavirin, amphotericin, TMP-SMX, pentamidine, rifabutin. TMP-SMX given at doses used for PCP prophylaxis rarely is the sole cause of neutropenia; if neutropenia does not improve after a trial of an alternative prophylactic regimen, TMP-SMX can be restarted.

c. **Infections.** MAC, CMV, disseminated fungal diseases (e.g., histoplasmosis)

2. **Treatment.** Only indicated if ANC is consistently < 750/mm^3 (some experts cite 500/mm^3). After underlying causes are corrected, consider G-CSF (Neupogen) 150-300 mcg (SQ) every 1-7 days. Start with 3x/week dosing, then titrate dose to maintain ANC > 1000/mm^3.

D. Eosinophilia

1. **Etiology**
   a. **Direct effect of HIV.** Sometimes seen with no apparent cause, especially in advanced HIV disease
   b. **Drug allergy.** Most commonly to TMP-SMX and other sulfonamides
   c. **Parasitic infection (rare).** Most HIV-related parasitic infections (e.g., toxoplasmosis, cryptosporidiosis, etc.) do not cause eosinophilia. Rare exceptions include *Isospora belli* and strongyloidiasis (if patient from endemic area)
2. **Treatment.** Consider withdrawal of offending agent if associated with other allergic phenomena. Check stool for ova and parasites, strongyloides serology.

ONCOLOGIC COMPLICATIONS

Malignancies definitely associated with HIV infection include Kaposi's sarcoma, non-Hodkgin's lymphoma, Hodgkin's Disease, squamous cell neoplasia, and leiomyosarcoma (in children). Possible associated malignancies include seminoma, lung cancer, and multiple myeloma.

A. Kaposi's Sarcoma. Infection with HHV-8 is a critical viral cofactor; interaction between host immunosuppression, genetic factors, and this virus determine a patient's risk. In North America, Australia, and Western Europe, Kaposi's sarcoma occurs most commonly in gay/bisexual men. The incidence has diminished markedly since the introduction of potent antiretroviral therapy. In developing countries (especially in certain parts of Africa), Kaposi's sarcoma is more evenly distributed among men and women.

1. **Presentation.** Usually presents as violaceous nodules and plaques on the skin; oral cavity and other mucosal surfaces may be involved. With more advanced immunosuppression, visceral involvement (lungs, gastrointestinal tract) can be life-threatening. Invasion of local lymphatics can lead to chronic

edema of the limbs, face, and genitals, with increased risk of bacterial superinfection.

2. **Treatment.** Initiation of antiretroviral therapy is often sufficient to cause regression of disease. For disease that progresses despite antivirals, options include local measures (intralesional chemotherapy, radiation therapy) and systemic chemotherapy (liposomal anthracyclines are especially effective).

B. **Non-Hodgkin's Lymphoma (NHL).** In patients with HIV infection, NHL is most commonly a manifestation of advanced immunosuppression (CD4 < $100/mm^3$).

1. **Presentation.** Clinical presentation reflects extranodal involvement of the disease: typically, gastrointestinal tract (45%), bone marrow (20%), and CNS (20-30%). Often multiple sites are involved simultaneously. Of note, the patient with AIDS who has diffuse adenopathy and fever will more likely have a systemic infection (most commonly *M. avium* complex, histoplasmososis, cryptococcus) rather than lymphoma. Although the incidence of NHL has declined since the introduction of potent antiretroviral therapy, it has done so to a lesser degree than other opportunistic infections. As a result, NHL in some centers is responsible for a higher proportion of AIDS-related complications compared with the pre-antiretroviral era.
2. **Treatment.** Generally involves full-dose chemotherapy (e.g., CHOP), with use of recombinant growth factors (G-CSF, erythropoietin) as needed to support cell lines. Initiation of antiretroviral therapy concurrently with chemotherapy may improve outcome by reducing infectious complications and improving recovery time of bone marrow function. It is important to avoid the use of antiviral agents that may have overlapping toxicities with the prescribed chemotherapy (e.g., avoid d4T or ddI when patients are receiving systemic vincristine therapy, as this increases the risk of peripheral neuropathy; avoid ZDV since this may further suppress the bone marrow).

C. **Primary CNS Lymphoma.** Usually a manifestation of advanced HIV disease, with the vast majority of patients having a CD4 cell count < $50/mm^3$.

1. **Presentation.** The typical presentation is one of focal neurologic deficits or seizures, reflecting focal lesion(s) in the brain. MRI findings typically show lesions with irregular enhancement, sometimes involving the corpus callosum and crossing the midline; mass effect is generally evident. Appearance of primary CNS lymphoma is similar to that of CNS toxoplasmosis; in the latter, lesions are often greater in number, but radiographic abnormalities overlap significantly.
2. **Diagnosis.** If a patient with advanced AIDS presents with focal enhancing lesion(s) on MRI or CT scan and is either toxoplasmosis seronegative or taking TMP-SMX for toxoplasmosis prophylaxis, then primary CNS lymphoma is the most likely diagnosis. While noninvasive testing such as thallium SPECT scan, PET scan, and CSF studies for cytology and Epstein-Barr virus DNA (by

PCR) can sometimes be helpful, the definitive diagnosis is generally made through stereotactic brain biopsy.

3. **Treatment.** The prognosis of primary CNS lymphoma remains quite poor, especially for patients who fail antiretroviral therapy. Treatment with steroids and radiation therapy is palliative. Rare patients have experienced sustained remissions after initiating antiretroviral therapy and achieving a significant improvement in immune function.

D. **Cervical Cancer.** Compared to HIV-negative women, the incidence of cervical cancer in HIV-infected women is higher and the disease may be more aggressive. Cervical cancer is strongly associated with HPV infection and progressive immunosuppression. A diagnosis of cervical cancer along with a positive HIV serology is considered AIDS defining. Recommendations for screening include a Pap smear twice the first year after HIV diagnosis, and yearly thereafter if normal. This strategy is associated with a low risk of invasive cervical cancer, comparable to HIV-negative women.

E. **Anal Cancer.** The incidence of anal cancer in gay men is approximately 80 times that of the general population. As with cervical cancer, anal cancer is strongly associated with HPV infection. Although screening for anal cancer using anal Pap smears could identify precancerous lesions much as with cervical cancer, guidelines for screening have not been incorporated into formal recommendations. Pending these recommendations, a reasonable strategy is as follows:

1. At a minimum, perform annual periodic visual inspection and a digital rectal exam.
2. Perform anal Pap smear for any anorectal complaints; some recommend annual testing on all HIV-positive gay men.
3. For low-grade squamous intraepithelial lesion (SIL), repeat screening in 6-12 months; for high-grade lesions, refer to a colorectal surgeon for anoscopy and/or anal colposcopy with biopsy.

ENDOCRINE COMPLICATIONS

A. **Adrenal Insufficiency.** Although adrenal gland involvement has been documented in up to two-thirds of patients with AIDS on postmortem examination, clinically relevant adrenal insufficiency is rare (~ 3% of patients with AIDS) and is generally a manifestation of late-stage AIDS.

1. **Etiology.** Potential causes of primary adrenal dysfunction include destruction of the adrenal gland from opportunistic infections (especially CMV), neoplasms (Kaposi's sarcoma, lymphoma), hemorrhage, and infarction. More commonly, adrenal insufficiency results from the adverse

effect of medications, including ketoconazole (decreased steroidogenesis), rifampin/rifabutin (enhanced cortisol metabolism), and corticosteroids/megestrol acetate (suppressed pituitary secretion of corticotropin due to intrinsic glucocorticoid activity; latter may actually induce Cushing syndrome with prolonged use). An important recently identified cause of cortisol excess is the use of inhaled steroids (esp. fluticasone) with ritonavir. Ritonavir blocks the metabolism of many corticosteroids, leading to increased exposure and iatrogenic Cushing's syndrome. Conversely, stopping the inhaled steroid can cause adrenal insufficiency (J Clin Endocrinol Metab 2005;90:4394-8).

2. **Diagnosis.** Adrenal insufficiency should be suspected in a patient with advanced HIV disease or recent therapy with steroid-interfering medications who presents with hypotension, profound weakness, or electrolyte abnormalities (hyponatremia, hyperkalemia). Evaluation consists of measurement of a.m. cortisol; if normal and the diagnosis is still suspected, perform a corticotropin stimulation test. If the diagnosis is still suspected despite a normal corticotropin stimulation test, referral to an endocrinologist is warranted since some patients with AIDS have peripheral resistance to glucocorticoid action.
3. **Treatment.** Patients with basal low cortisol levels, even if asymptomatic, require life-long replacement therapy (prednisone 5 mg [PO] at bedtime). For corticotropin hyporesponsiveness, steroid supplementation for stressing conditions (e.g., surgery, intercurrent illness) is indicated. For life-threatening situations, immediate treatment with dexamethasone 4 mg (IV) is indicated; this will not impair the diagnostic utility of the corticotropin stimulation test.

B. **Hypogonadism.** Men with HIV infection are more likely to be hypogonadal than HIV-negative controls. The frequency of this abnormality increases with progressive immunodeficiency and may reach 50% in patients with AIDS. In general, there is no detectable underlying etiology. HIV-related hypogonadism is associated with weakness, weight loss, decreased libido, and impaired quality of life. Replacement therapy can improve many of these symptoms, especially when combined with a resistance exercise program. While low testosterone levels have also been observed in HIV-infected women, replacement therapy is experimental. Treatment for men consists of testosterone gel (Androgel) 5 mg q24h or injectable testosterone cypionate/enanthate 200 mg every other week. Potential side effects include acne, gynecomastia, and testicular atrophy. Monitor prostate specific antigen annually for patients on replacement therapy.

C. **Thyroid Disease.** The thyroid gland is rarely involved in disseminated opportunistic infections (e.g., extrapulmonary pneumocystis). Chronically ill patients with HIV may have low T3, but TSH is generally normal. Immune response to antiretroviral therapy may unmask subclinical Grave's disease, leading to clinical hyperthyroidism. Treatment of Grave's disease consists of radioactive thyroid ablation or an anti-thyroid medication (e.g., methimazole) as directed by an endocrinologist. Beta-blockers can be used to ameliorate the symptoms of hyperthyroidism.

D. Pancreatitis. Clinical presentation is similar to HIV-negative patients, with nausea, vomiting, abdominal pain.

1. **Etiology**
   a. **Medications:** Common: ddI (increased risk with higher doses, hydroxyurea, alcohol use), d4T (risk especially high when d4T and ddI are prescribed together), pentamidine, corticosteroids . Less common: other NRTI's, TMP-SMX, protease inhibitors (when accompanied by very high triglyceride levels), INH, erythromycin.
   b. **Opportunistic infections.** Most commonly identified opportunistic infection to cause pancreatitis is CMV. Can rarely be caused by TB, MAC, intestinal protozoa (cryptosporidia, microsporidia), widely disseminated toxoplasmosis.
   c. **Non-HIV–related.** Alcohol, obesity, gallstones.
2. **Treatment.** Discontinue potentially offending drug; treat identified cause.

E. Hyperglycemia. Patients with HIV appear to be at higher risk of developing insulin resistance and diabetes mellitus than HIV-negative controls. Potential contributing factors include lipodystrophy syndrome (especially subcutaneous fat loss) and medications (especially certain PI-containing regimens, most notably indinavir).

1. **Diagnosis.** For patients on antiretroviral therapy, monitor serum glucose every 3 months as part of safety labs. If elevated or abnormal, consider a fasting glucose, insulin level, and hemoglobin A1C. A fasting blood glucose > 126 mg/dL or a glucose level > 200 mg/dL two hours after administration of 75 gm of glucose is diagnostic of diabetes mellitus.
2. **Treatment.** If the patient is on a protease inhibitor and has an undetectable HIV RNA and no history of extensive NRTI resistance, consider substituting an NNRTI (e.g., efavirenz, nevirapine) for the protease inhibitor. Alternatively, there is evidence that atazanavir may be least likely to lead to insulin resistance among the PI's, and hence can be substituted for other protease inhibitors. Alternatively, there is evidence that atazanavir may be least likely to lead to insulin resistance, and hence can be substituted for other protease inhibitors. Abacavir has also been used in this setting, although NRTI resistance compromises virologic efficacy of this strategy. If the patient is not on a protease inhibitor and fasting hyperglycemia persists, follow established guidelines for treatment of diabetes mellitus in the general population, including weight loss, dietary modification, and exercise. When medical therapy is required, consider the use of insulin sensitizing agents such as metformin 500 mg (PO) q12h or pioglitazone 15-30 mg (PO) q24h. In small studies, metformin therapy in patients with HIV has led to

improvements in insulin sensitivity, reduction in waist circumference, and decreased blood pressure. Pioglitazone in one study improved insulin sensitivity and subcutaneous fat stores, and appears to be safer in HIV patients than rosiglitazone, which has been associated with hyperlipidemia.

F. **Hypoglycemia.** Pentamidine induces hypoglycemia by lysing pancreatic islet cells. Monitor fingerstick glucose levels daily while patients receive this therapy. Prolonged, repeated use of pentamidine may result in diabetes mellitus from insulin deficiency.

G. **Ovarian Complications.** Amenorrhea is common in women with advanced AIDS who have significant weight loss. Menses may resume with weight gain and improvement in clinical status accompanying antiretroviral therapy.

H. **Bone Disease**

1. **Osteonecrosis.** This complication has been reported in association with HIV infection since the late 1980s, but it appears to be more common since the introduction of effective antiretroviral therapy (J AIDS 2006;42:286-92). It is not clear if the increased incidence is due simply to prolonged survival, or to a direct toxic effect of antiretroviral medications. The most commonly involved sites are the femoral heads, followed by the humeral heads, femoral condyles, proximal tibia, and small bones of the hands and wrists. Most patients will have traditional underlying risk factors, such as a history of corticosteroid use, hyperlipidemia, alcohol abuse, or a hypercoagulable state. The relationship to any specific form of antiretroviral therapy has not been conclusively demonstrated.
   a. **Diagnosis.** Consider osteonecrosis in a patient with refractory hip pain, especially if there are underlying risk factors (see above). If plain film imaging is negative, proceed to MRI, which is more sensitive. Bilateral imaging is indicated since the disease is often bilateral.
   b. **Treatment.** Conservative management with physical therapy is recommended initially. If pain persists, refer to an orthopedic surgeon for consideration of hip stabilization/hip replacement.

2. **Osteoporosis.** Osteopenia and osteoporosis have been reported in 22-50% and 3-21% of patients receiving chronic antiretroviral therapy, respectively. Spontaneous fractures have also been reported, although the risk is low. As with osteonecrosis, the relationship between bone demineralization and a specific antiretroviral drug class has not been established.
   a. **Diagnosis.** Routine screening is not indicated. If other risk factors for loss of bone density are present, the appropriate screening test is regional DEXA scanning. Secondary causes of osteopenia and osteoporosis should be evaluated, including thyrotoxicosis, hyperparathyroidism, hypogonadism, weight loss, alcohol intake, and certain medications

(especially corticosteroids).

b. **Treatment.** All patients should receive adequate diet, and if needed, supplements of calcium and vitamin D. If osteoporosis is demonstrated on DEXA scan (t-score of –2.5 or lower), consider biphosphonate therapy.

GASTROINTESTINAL TRACT COMPLICATIONS

A. Anorexia

1. **Etiology.** Commonly associated with advanced HIV disease, possibly due to high cytokine (especially TNF) levels that correlate with high titer HIV RNA. Other causes include depression, medications, opportunistic infections (especially MAC), and lactic acidosis (related to mitochondrial toxicity).
2. **Treatment.** Megecetrol acetate (Megace) liquid suspension 400-800 mg (PO) q24h improves appetite, quality of life. Weight gain that results is generally fat, not lean body mass. Side effects include hypogonadism, DVT, gynecomastia. Megace has corticosteroid properties, and therefore can lead to Cushings-like state (prolonged use) or adrenal insufficiency (when drug is withdrawn). Dronabinol (Marinol) 2.5 mg q12h stimulates appetite and reduces nausea. Dronabinol is a synthetic delta-9-tetrahydrocannabinol (THC), the active ingredient in marijuana. The main side effect is oversedation. Patients should start with a dose at bedtime and then increase to q12h as tolerated.

B. Nausea/Vomiting

1. **Etiology**
   a. **Medications.** Direct effect of antiretroviral medications (especially PI's, ZDV, abacavir hypersensitivity), medication-related pancreatitis (see above), or lactic acidosis from NRTI's.
   b. **Opportunistic infections.** Intestinal protozoa (e.g., cryptosporidiosis, isospora, giardiasis – all usually accompanied by diarrhea), CMV esophagitis/gastritis, GI tract involvement of MAC.
   c. **Others.** Gastric lymphoma, CNS process producing mass effect (toxoplasmosis or lymphoma) or raised intracerebral pressure (cryptococcal meningitis).
2. **Treatment.** Address underlying etiology. If felt to be due to the direct effect of antiretrovirals, choose an alternate regimen if possible (e.g., substitute tenofovir for ZDV, efavirenz for PI). If underlying cause cannot be treated or removed, or for temporary relief of symptoms, therapeutic options include: prochlorperazine (Compazine) 10 mg (PO) or 25 mg (PR) q12h prn; metoclopramide (Reglan) 10 mg (PO) q6h prn; trimethobenzamide (Tigan) 250 mg (PO) q6h prn; lorazepam 0.5-1.0 mg (PO or IV) q6h prn; ondansetron (Zofran) 4-8 mg (PO) q8h prn or 32 mg (IV or IM) as a single

dose; dronabinol (Marinol) 2.5-5.0 mg (PO) q12h. Patients with HIV are at increased risk for phenothiazine-related dystonia, which may occur with prochlorperazine, metoclopramide, and trimethobenzamide. Treat dystonia with diphenhydramine (Benadryl) 50 mg (PO or IV) x 1 dose.

C. Diarrhea

1. Etiology

a. Infection. Acute diarrhea: salmonella, shigella, campylobacter, *C. difficile*, giardiasis, cyclospora; subacute/chronic diarrhea: giardiasis, cryptosporidia, microsporidia, isospora, CMV.

b. Medication-related. Especially nelfinavir, all ritonavir-boosted PI's, ritonavir, buffered version of ddI; can be part of abacavir hypersensitivity syndrome. Medication-related diarrhea is rarely associated with weight loss or fever (abacavir excluded).

2. Treatment. Treat underlying cause (see Chapter 5). If PI-related, consider changing to an alternative PI (e.g., atazanavir, indinavir) less likely to cause diarrhea, or to an NNRTI (efavirenz or nevirapine). To avoid resistance, NNRTI replacement should only be considered when the HIV RNA is < 50 copies/mL, and preferably when there is no history of treatment failure that would lead to NRTI resistance. If diarrhea persists or if medication changes are not possible, offer symptomatic therapy with psyllium 1 tsp q12h-24h, loperamide 2 mg q6h prn, calcium 500 mg q12h; pancreatic enzymes 1-2 tabs with each meal, Lomotil 1-2 tabs q8h prn, or octreotide 100-500 mcg (SQ) q12h.

D. Oral or Esophageal Ulcers

1. Presentation. Intensely painful ulcers of various size; esophageal ulcers cause severe dysphagia. May occur at any stage of HIV disease (including primary infection), but more common with progressive immunosuppression (CD4 < 100, associated neutropenia). Most common diagnosis is idiopathic aphthous ulcers; other major causes include CMV, HSV, histoplasmosis, lymphoma. For first-time presentation, culture for HSV and refer for biopsy to exclude other causes.

2. Treatment. For idiopathic aphthous ulcers, start with symptom relief, followed by application of local steroids, followed by either systemic steroids or thalidomide. Lesions sometimes respond to immune reconstitution from antiretroviral therapy along with resolution of neutropenia (adjunctive therapy with G-CSF may hasten healing). Therapeutic modalities include:

a. Symptom reduction with viscous lidocaine (2%)

b. Topical fluocinonide (Lidex) 0.05% ointment mixed 1:1 with Orobase; apply q6h as needed

c. Dexamethasone 0.5/5M elixir mouth rinse q8h-12h

d. Local corticosteroid injections by oral surgeon

e. Prednisone 40-60 mg/day x 1-2 weeks, tapered as tolerated over 1-2 weeks or longer as needed

f. Thalidomide 200 mg (PO) at bedtime x 4-6 weeks, followed by 100 mg (PO) at bedtime twice weekly. Side effects include sedation, constipation, peripheral neuropathy. Severe teratogenicity of thalidomide requires that physicians register with company-sponsored monitoring program before prescribing (see http://www.celgene.com/steps/index.htm). Women of childbearing age must use at least two forms of contraception and have regular pregnancy tests while receiving thalidomide. Informed consent in package insert must be signed before therapy is initiated.

E. HIV Cholangiopathy

1. **Presentation.** Presents with right upper quadrant pain, fever, and sometimes jaundice. Laboratory evaluation invariably demonstrates increased alkaline phosphatase. Generally occurs with severe immunosuppression (CD4 < 100/mm^3). Imaging with ultrasound or ERCP shows dilated or prominent intrahepatic and extrahepatic ducts. Papillary stenosis may also be present.
2. **Etiology.** Differential diagnosis include cholelithiasis, acalculous cholecystitis, infiltrative infectious or neoplastic diseases of the liver. Screen for infectious etiology, including stool for ova/parasites and/or ERCP aspirates for cryptosporidia, microsporidia, cyclospora, CMV.
3. **Treatment.** Symptomatic improvement is sometimes seen with endoscopic-guided sphincterotomy or stenting. Treat underlying infectious process, if identified.

RENAL COMPLICATIONS

A. HIV-Associated Nephropathy. A form of progressive glomerulosclerosis, leading to massive proteinuria and progressive renal dysfunction. Over 80% of cases occur in blacks. Renal biopsy shows extensive collapsing glomerulosclerosis, tubular ectasia, and tubulo-interstitial disease. Occurs most commonly with low CD4 cell counts (<100/mm^3), but may occur at any level of immunosuppression. Very uncommon with undetectable HIV RNA (Clin Infect Dis 2006;43:377-80).

1. **Presentation.** Clinical presentation varies from asymptomatic to symptoms of hypoalbuminemia and renal failure (edema, fatigue, anemia). Hypertension generally is absent. Renal ultrasound demonstrates enlarged or normal-sized kidneys. The cardinal laboratory feature is proteinuria > 1 gm/day, usually with rapidly progressive renal failure evolving over weeks to months to end-stage renal disease requiring dialysis.
2. **Diagnostic Considerations.** Biopsy should be considered to rule out other causes of progressive renal disease, such as HCV-associated renal disease, medication-associated toxicity (see below), or a non-HIV-related cause.

3. **Treatment.** Effective options include antiretroviral therapy (case reports suggest PI-based therapy may lead to resolution of disease), ACE inhibitors, and high-dose corticosteroids (60 mg prednisone q24h x 1 month followed by gradual taper) (Kidney International 2000;58:1253). Since high-dose steroids are associated with further immune suppression and other complications, a reasonable approach is to begin with antiretroviral therapy plus an ACE inhibitor (e.g., captopril 6.25 mg q8h).

B. **Medication-Related Renal Disease.** HIV-related medications most likely to cause nephrotoxicity are listed below. (See antiretroviral drug summaries in Chapter 9 for dosing in renal insufficiency.)

1. **Indinavir.** Can crystalize in urine, leading to a variety of renal conditions, including nephrolithiasis, crystal-related nephropathy, and sterile pyuria. Risk may be dose-related and is more common when indinavir is dosed with ritonavir as a PK booster. Risk can be reduced by ingestion of at least 1.5 liters of water daily. For acute renal colic, a trial of increasing oral hydration is warranted, after which, IV hydration and cessation of indinavir and other antiretroviral medications is recommended until the condition resolves. For severe nephrolithiasis or other renal complication of indinavir, consider alternative antiretroviral therapy. If no other options exist, the dose of indinavir should be modified.
2. **Pentamidine.** Can cause renal failure in up to 50% of patients; other adverse effects include electrolyte/mineral wasting and hypoglycemia. Risk is related to cumulative dose; monitor creatinine, electrolytes, glucose, calcium, and phosphate during therapy.
3. **Foscarnet.** Induces dose-related renal failure as well as wasting of potassium, calcium, and phosphate. Dose adjustment is necessary for reduced creatinine clearance. Supplement potassium, calcium, and phosphorus as needed.
4. **Cidofovir.** Associated with dose-related renal toxicity, which can be reduced by concomitant administration of probenecid and hydration. Check serum creatinine and urine for protein prior to each dose; if creatinine is > 2 gm/dL or there is more than 2+ proteinuria, do not administer further cidofovir as renal toxicity may be irreversible.
5. **Tenofovir.** Can rarely cause tubular injury, leading to increased creatinine. Sometimes accompanied by Fanconi's syndrome, with phosphate wasting and acidosis. Renal toxicity is more likely to occur in those with underlying renal disease or advanced HIV infection (Clin Infect Dis 2005;15:1194-8, J Infect Dis 2008;197:102). Use calculated creatinine clearance (Cockgroft-Gault equation) to assess renal function, and reduce dose based on degree of renal insufficiency as recommended in the package insert.
6. **Amphotericin B.** Dose-dependent renal toxicity is common. Liposomal preparations are less nephrotoxic.
7. **Trimethoprim-sulfamethoxazole (TMP-SMX).** May cause hyperkalemia

through amiloride-like effect from trimethoprim, especially when used at high doses for PCP treatment. Sulfonamide component can rarely cause crystal nephropathy (reversible with hydration).

8. **Acyclovir.** High-dose IV administration can crystalize in kidney and cause acute renal failure. Risk can be reduced with adequate hydration, and renal dysfunction usually responds to hydration and cessation of drug.

C. **HCV-Associated Renal Disease.** Often a manifestation of HCV-associated mixed cryoglobulinemia.
   1. **Presentation.** Patients may present with palpable purpura or other dermatologic signs, along with hematuria, proteinuria, and sometimes renal failure. Other related laboratory findings include HCV RNA in plasma, cryoglobulins in blood, and low complement; renal biopsy shows HCV-related immune complexes.
   2. **Treatment.** Therapy directed at hepatitis C (PEG-interferon plus ribavirin) can lead to improvement in renal disease and other manifestations of cryoglobulinemia.

D. **Heroin Nephropathy.** Can coexist with other forms of renal failure listed above. Results from glomerular injury, presumably from toxic effects of heroin or other contaminants. Distinguished from HIV-associated nephropathy by a slower rate of progression, small (as opposed to large) kidneys on ultrasound, and less proteinuria. Treatment consists of cessation of drug use.

CARDIAC COMPLICATIONS

A. **HIV-Related Cardiomyopathy** (JAMA 2008;299:324-31). Biventricular reduction in ejection fraction, with pathologic features typical of myocarditis and/or immune-mediated cardiomyopathy. Prevalence varies widely depending on definition; echocardiogram may show reduced ejection fraction in up to 50% of patients with AIDS, but symptomatic cardiomyopathy occurs in only 1-3%. More common with progressive immunodeficiency, especially when CD4 cell count < 100.
   1. **Etiology.** Usually idiopathic. Differential diagnosis includes several causes, not mutually exclusive: HIV itself, secondary infection (CMV, toxoplasmosis, coxsackie, adenovirus, Chagas), disordered immune response leading to autoimmune myocarditis, nutritional deficiencies (selenium, carnitine), drug toxicity (NRTI-associated mitochondrial toxicity, alcohol, doxorubicin).
   2. **Presentation.** Presents as left ventricular failure, with dyspnea, congestive heart failure, elevated jugular venous pressure, a prominent S_3 on exam. Chest x-ray typically demonstrates an enlarged heart, and echocardiogram shows marked biventricular dysfunction with reduced ejection fraction.

Diagnosis is made after exclusion of other common causes of low EF (alcohol, poor nutrition, myocardial ischemia). Cardiac biopsy is rarely useful.

3. **Treatment.** Patients should receive antiretroviral therapy plus usual therapies for heart failure (diuretics, beta-blockers, ACE inhibitors are often quite effective in reducing symptoms). For manifestations of disseminated CMV disease or a positive blood CMV viral load, empiric CMV treatment with valganciclovir 900 mg (PO) q12h x 3 weeks. Although case reports have shown improvement in ejection fraction after cessation of NRTI's, this is a much less common cause of cardiomyopathy than HIV itself. If cardiomyopathy occurs while a patient is on NRTI's – especially if HIV RNA is low and CD4 cell count > 200/mm^3 – it is reasonable to discontinue NRTI's for 1-2 months to assess whether improvement in cardiac function occurs.

B. Pericarditis/Pericardial Effusion

1. **Etiology.** Pericardial fluid may be due to HIV itself or a complicating malignancy/opportunistic infection. The most common malignancy is lymphoma, where an effusion may be the first manifestation of an extranodal high-grade B-cell lymphoma; Kaposi's sarcoma causes effusions generally only when the disease is widespread elsewhere. In addition, numerous common and opportunistic infections have been reported to cause pericarditis in HIV patients, including pyogenic bacteria (especially *S. aureus* and *S. pneumoniae*), TB, atypical mycobacteria, cryptococcal disease, disseminated histoplasmosis, and CMV.
2. **Presentation and Diagnosis.** Often diagnosed incidentally through enlarged cardiac silhouette and subsequent echocardiogram. May be asymptomatic or cause chest pain, dyspnea, cardiac tamponade, pericardial friction rub. Pericardiocentesis is indicated for large or symptomatic effusions, with fluid sent for cultures (routine, fungal, mycobacterial) and cytology.
3. **Treatment.** Directed at underlying condition. If idiopathic pericarditis, consider starting antiretroviral therapy, and manage symptoms with NSAIDs and corticosteroids (as in HIV-negative patients).

C. Tricuspid Valve Endocarditis

1. **Etiology.** Injection drug users (IDUs) with HIV, particularly those with lower CD4 cell counts, are at substantially higher risk for endocarditis than HIV-negative IDUs (J Infect Dis 2002;185:1761-6). *Staphylococcus aureus* is the most common pathogen. In one series, rates of infection included *S. aureus* (73%), coagulase-negative *Staphylococcus* species (1%), *Staphylococcus* species not otherwise classified (7%), *Streptococcus* species (13%), *Pseudomonas* species (2%), *Bacillus* species (2%), and other organisms (2%). Most urban centers are experiencing an increasing rate of MRSA.
2. **Presentation and Diagnosis.** Patients typically present with fever, weight loss, and sometimes pulmonary symptoms (dyspnea, chest pain) reflective

of septic emboli arising from an infected tricuspid valve. Physical examination usually reveals a heart murmur ± evidence of peripheral septic emboli. Chest x-ray may show multiple septic emboli, some with cavitation. An echocardiogram should be performed to assess for valvular vegetations. Diagnosis is confirmed when a patient with the above clinical presentation has positive blood cultures for an organism known to be associated with endocarditis.

3. **Treatment.** While a short-course (2 weeks) of therapy has been effective in HIV-negative IDUs with tricuspid endocarditis, this regimen cannot be recommended in HIV-positive patients. Recommended regimens include:
   - Methicillin-sensitive S. aureus: Nafcillin 2 gm (IV) q4h x 28 days plus gentamicin 1 mg/kg (IV) q8h x 3-5 days or until blood cultures clear
   - Methicillin-resistant S. aureus or beta-lactam allergy: Vancomycin 1 gm (IV) q12h x 28 days plus gentamicin 1 mg/kg (IV) q8h x 3-5 days or until blood cultures clear. Alternative to vancomycin is daptomycin (IV) 6 mg/kg q24h x 4 weeks
   - Unable or unwilling to receive IV therapy: Ciprofloxacin 750 mg (PO) q12h plus rifampin 300 mg (PO) q12h x 4 weeks. This regimen cannot be used with PI's due to rifampin-PI interaction. Linezolid 600 mg (PO) q12h x 4 weeks can be used as an alternative (limited data)

PULMONARY COMPLICATIONS

A. **Pulmonary Hypertension** (see also JAMA 2008; 299:324-31). Idiopathic elevation of pulmonary pressures is sometimes seen in HIV infection. The pathological process is similar to primary pulmonary hypertension (i.e., hypertrophy of vascular endothelium). Pulmonary hypertension is more common in women and can occur at any CD4 cell count.

1. **Presentation.** Dyspnea on exertion, palpitations, chest pain. Exam may reveal elevated JVP and precordial heave. Diagnosis is supported by echocardiogram and doppler studies showing right ventricular hypertrophy and elevated PA pressures. Most sensitive test is right heart catheterization, where pressures will exceed 30 mmHg. Recurrent pulmonary emboli should be excluded as a possible cause.
2. **Treatment.** Epoprostenol (FloLan) by continuous infusion. Requires placement of a permanent central venous catheter. Diuretics also help relieve symptoms. Anticoagulation is generally indicated. Sildenafil is being investigated as a possible adjunct to therapy. There are mixed reports on whether antiretroviral therapy improves hemodynamics or outcome.

B. **Lymphocytic Interstitial Pneumonitis (LIP).** An idiopathic form of diffuse lung disease that is more common in children. Tends to occur with moderate immunosuppression (CD4 cell count 200-400/mm^3) and mimics PCP.

1. **Presentation and Diagnosis.** Cough, dyspnea on exertion, exercise oxygen desaturation. Usually afebrile. Chest x-ray and chest CT show diffuse bilateral reticulonodular infiltrates. Differentiated from PCP by generally higher CD4 cell counts and lower LDH. Diagnosed by bronchioalveolar lavage (BAL) with biopsy, which will exclude PCP and yield the characteristic histopathology of LIP (patchy lymphocytic infiltration and no microorganisms on special stains).
2. **Treatment.** Antiretroviral therapy can either improve LIP or worsen it through enhanced immune activity. Prednisone usually achieves rapid reduction in dyspnea, but tapering dose may be accompanied by a relapse of symptoms.

C. **Emphysema.** Cigarette smoking is associated with a more rapid progression to bullous emphysema in patients with HIV compared to HIV-negative controls. Clinical presentation and treatment are the same as for the general population.

D. **Pulmonary Kaposi's Sarcoma.** Generally occurs only in patients with advanced HIV disease and extensive Kaposi's sarcoma elsewhere.

1. **Presentation and Diagnosis.** Chest x-ray demonstrates nodules, masses, and/or pleural effusions. Diagnosed by visual inspection of the airway during bronchoscopy, where typical violaceous plaques may be observed.
2. **Treatment.** Antiretroviral therapy may lead to dramatic improvement in even severe Kaposi's sarcoma, although temporary flares due to immune reconstitution have been reported. Concomitant systemic chemotherapy is also generally required.

HEENT COMPLICATIONS

A. **Aphthous Ulcers.** See p. 110.

B. **Oral Hairy Leukoplakia**

1. **Presentation.** Presents as ribbed, "corduroy"-like white patches on the side of the tongue. More common with increased immunosuppression (CD4 < 200/mm^3). Usually painless. Distinguished from oral thrush in that oral hairy leukoplakia does not rub off with tongue depressor. Caused by Epstein-Barr virus.
2. **Treatment.** No treatment is needed unless the patient is symptomatic. If treatment is desired, antiretroviral therapy often leads to resolution. Other treatment options include acyclovir 800 mg (PO) 5x/day or famciclovir 500 mg (PO) q12h or valacyclovir 1000 mg (PO) q8h until resolution. Topical application of podophyllin is sometimes effective.

C. Salivary Gland Enlargement

1. **Presentation.** Can occur at any stage of HIV infection and usually worsens with disease progression. Often accompanied by xerostomia. Biopsy shows lymphoid infiltration, possibly due to HIV itself. A CT scan is recommended to differentiate solid from cystic enlargement. Differential diagnosis includes infectious parotitis, which presents more acutely with fever and local pain.
2. **Treatment.** Antiretroviral therapy is the preferred approach. Other forms of treatment include repeated aspiration of fluid-filled cysts when symptomatic, local measures for dry mouth (sugarless gum, artificial saliva), and prednisone 40 mg (PO) q24h x 1 week followed by gradual taper over 1-2 weeks.

D. Lymphoepithelial Cysts

1. **Presentation.** Presents as enlarged cervical cysts that can mimic lymphadenopathy. Can occur at any CD4 cell count. A biopsy is needed to rule out lymphoma, opportunistic infections. Cause is unknown.
2. **Treatment.** Antiretroviral therapy often causes dramatic reduction in size of cysts.

E. Gingivitis/Periodontitis

1. **Presentation.** Presents as painful gums with easy bleeding, along with erythematous and receding gingiva. May be the initial manifestation of underlying HIV disease. Severity correlates with stage of immunosuppression. Caused by oral anaerobic bacteria (usually polymicrobial), and exacerbated by poor local oral hygiene, smoking, alcoholism.
2. **Treatment.** Improve local hygiene, (brush, floss, antibacterial mouth rinse). Curettage by dentist/periodontist may be helpful. For severe cases, treat for 7-10 days with metronidazole 500 mg (PO) q8h or clindamycin 300 mg (PO) q6h or amoxicillin-clavulanate 850 mg (PO) q12h.

MUSCULOSKELETAL COMPLICATIONS

A. HIV Arthropathy

1. **Presentation.** Presents as painful arthropathy, often involving multiple joints. Pain out of proportion to physical findings. Cause is unknown.
2. **Treatment.** NSAIDs, other pain relievers.

B. Reiter's Syndrome

1. **Presentation.** Asymmetrical polyarthritis involving the large joints of lower extremities. Arthritis is seen in conjunction with urethritis, skin lesions (circinate balanitis, keratoderma blennorrhagica), ocular disease. May also

occur after gastroenteritis. Appears to occur with greater frequency among HIV patients, usually in association with HLA-B27.

2. **Diagnosis.** Differential diagnosis includes septic arthritis; if joint effusions are present, arthrocentesis with cultures/gram stain is indicated. Urethral swab for chlamydia and gonorrhea is also recommended.
3. **Treatment.** Consider treatment of urethritis with empiric chlamydia therapy with azithromycin 1 gm (PO) x 1 dose. Other measures include NSAIDs and referral to rheumatology for possible immunosuppressive therapy (prednisone, methotrexate, TNF antagonists).

C. **Pyomyositis.** Focal infection of muscle often occurring at site of injections, trauma.

1. **Presentation.** Presents as localized pain, swelling, fever. Usually caused by *Staphylococcus aureus* (less commonly with other pyogenic bacteria, e.g., streptococci, gram negative rods). More common with advanced HIV immunosuppression (CD4 cell count < 100).
2. **Diagnosis.** Imaging of suspected area with CT followed by diagnostic aspiration for gram stain/culture.
3. **Treatment.** Antibiotics directed at causative pathogen (usually an anti-staphylococcal penicillin or vancomycin). May also require surgical incision/drainage.

NEUROLOGIC COMPLICATIONS

A. **Distal Sensory Neuropathy.** Caused by HIV itself and/or neurotoxic effects of medications, in particular the di-deoxy NRTI's (d4T, ddI, ddC).

1. **Presentation.** Typically presents as pain, aching, burning, or tingling of the distal extremities (toes/feet more commonly than fingers/hands). Pain is often worse at night. Principal risk factors include the stage of HIV disease and exposure to the above listed drugs, especially when used in combination.
2. **Diagnosis and Evaluation.** Usually clinical, based on patient history. Reduced pin-prick and vibration sense in the involved extremities support the diagnosis, but symptoms often precede objective physical findings. Attempt to identify contributing/other causes, including B_{12} deficiency, syphilis, CMV, other neurotoxic agents (dapsone, INH, vincristine; avoid using these drugs if possible with d4T or ddI). If presentation is confusing, refer for EMG and nerve conduction studies, which will show an axonal neuropathy.
3. **Treatment.** Withdraw offending agents, in particular d4T and ddI; symptoms may persist or even worsen for several weeks after cessation of these drugs, and severe neuropathy may be irreversible. Antiretroviral therapy should be continued and one of several therapies used for

neuropathic symptoms can be administered:

- NSAID's or acetaminophen for mild pain
- Avoid tight-fitting shoes, extremes of temperature
- Gabapentin 300 mg at bedtime; increase up to 1200 mg divided q6-8h as needed
- Nortriptyline 10 mg at bedtime; increase up to 75 mg at bedtime as tolerated
- Lamictal 25 mg q12h; increase up to 150 mg q12h as tolerated.
- Topical therapy: capsaicin (may make symptoms worse), lidocaine patches
- Acupuncture
- Severe pain may require chronic long-acting narcotic pain relievers (e.g., methadone, MS-Contin, transdermal fentanyl).

B. Other Forms of Neuropathy

1. Types

a. **Acute inflammatory demyelinating neuropathy (AIDP, Guillan-Barre syndrome).** Ascending motor weakness usually without sensory involvement. Reported in early and late stage HIV. May evolve into a chronic form with waxing and waning symptoms. Treatment consists of steroids, plasmapheresis, IVIG. Prognosis is variable for all–tends to be best for mononeuritis especially if due to acute HIV infection.

b. **Mononeuritis multiplex.** Scattered, asymmetrical, motor and sensory deficits (e.g., facial weakness, foot drop). Reported in acute and chronic HIV. Some cases ascribed to CMV in advanced HIV (CD4 < $50/mm^3$). Treatment consists of steroids, IVIG. If caused by CMV, treat with valganciclovir at standard doses.

c. **HIV-associated neuromuscular weakness syndrome.** Rare complication of NRTI-therapy (especially d4T), presenting as progressive ascending paralysis in association with lactic acidosis. When severe, mechanical ventilation may be required. Treatment consist of withdrawal of NRTI's, especially d4T. Residual neurologic impairment is common after recovery.

d. **Progressive polyradiculopathy.** Complication of advanced HIV disease that typically presents with lower extremity weakness, anaesthesia in a "saddle" distribution (perineal area), and/or bowel and bladder dysfunction. Most common causes include CMV polyradiculitis (p. 71) and lymphoma. Diagnostically, obtain an MRI of the lumbosacral spine to exclude a mass lesion, then proceed to CSF exam. If due to CMV, the usual CSF finding is increased WBC (predominantly polys), increased protein, and positive CMV PCR. If due to lymphoma, the CSF shows increased protein and lymphoma cells on cytology. For CMV polyradiculitis, treat x 3-4 weeks or until improvement with either ganciclovir 5 mg/kg (IV) q12h or valganciclovir 900 mg (PO) q12h or foscarnet 90 mg/kg (IV) q12h; for severe cases, some advocate ganciclovir plus foscarnet. For lymphoma, treat with chemotherapy plus radiation.

2. **Prognosis.** Prognosis is variable for all forms of neuropathy but tends to be best for mononeuritis, especially if due to acute HIV infection.

C. **HIV-Associated Dementia (AIDS dementia, HIV encephalitis/encephalopathy).** Typical presentation at onset consists of short-term memory loss, often with apathy or withdrawal from usual activities. As the disease progresses, cognitive impairment worsens, and speech, motor, and gait disturbances develop. Seizures and akinetic mutism are late-stage manifestations. The incidence of this complication has decreased dramatically since the widespread introduction of combination antiretroviral therapy in 1996. Progression of dementia is gradual (usually over months) and can be arrested/reversed with potent antiretroviral therapy. A more rapidly-progressive form has also been reported. HIV dementia almost always occurs in the late stages of HIV disease (CD4 < $100/mm^3$, HIV RNA > 100,000 copies/mL), but on rare occasions occurs with relatively preserved immune function and low plasma HIV RNA. In the latter case, relatively high HIV RNA levels are often present in the CSF.

1. **Diagnosis.** Diagnosis is based on a combination of clinical, laboratory, and imaging criteria, as well as exclusion of alternative causes (depression, adverse drug effects, neurosyphilis, CMV encephalitis). HIV-associated dementia should be suspected in a patient with advanced HIV disease and subacute to chronic cognitive impairment, especially short-term memory loss. Administration of the four-step HIV-dementia scale (AIDS Reader 2002;12:29) may help quantify the extent of deficits. MRI shows cerebral atrophy and often non-enhancing white matter abnormalities that can be indistinguishable from progressive multifocal leukoencephalopathy (PML). CSF exam is usually abnormal, with elevated protein and low-level lymphocytic pleocytosis. When HIV RNA in the CSF is measured, it is usually detectable at 1000 copies/mL or higher; an undetectable CSF HIV RNA is unusual in HIV dementia and suggests an alternative diagnosis.
2. **Treatment.** Potent antiretroviral therapy is the mainstay of therapy and can lead to dramatic improvement, especially in treatment-naïve individuals. Selection of drugs with higher penetration into the CNS is theoretically preferable, although there are no definitive clinical data to support this approach over choosing alternative agents. Antiretroviral agents with the best CSF penetration are ZDV, ABC, d4T, NVP, IDV; somewhat lower penetration occurs with ddI, 3TC, EFV, LPV, FPV. An appropriate initial regimen could consist of ZDV/3TC (Combivir) 1 (PO) q12h plus nevirapine 200 mg (PO) q12h (after 14 days of 200 mg q24h) plus indinavir 800 mg q12h plus ritonavir 100-200 mg (PO) q12h. In a patient who has failed antiretroviral therapy, treatment is based on blood resistance testing to maximize antiviral potency.

PSYCHIATRIC COMPLICATIONS

Psychiatric illness is more common in patients with HIV than in those with other medical illnesses of comparable severity. Potential explanations include pre-existing psychiatric illness which predisposes to high-risk behavior for HIV acquisition (substance abuse, sexual addiction), extreme grief reactions from having a stigmatized illness, or neurotoxic effects of HIV manifesting as psychiatric illness. For all psychiatric illnesses, consider starting antiretroviral therapy even if there are otherwise no indications, as therapy is associated with improved neuropsychiatric function. Carefully review package inserts and drug interaction tables at www.aidsinfo.nih.gov prior to prescribing any psychotropic agent.

A. Depression

1. **Presentation and Diagnosis.** Common symptoms include depressed mood, decreased interest in work/leisure activities, blunted affect, sleep disturbances, alterations in appetite, forgetfulness, and diminished concentration. Key differential is HIV dementia, but depressed mood is usually not a prominent feature of dementia. Be sure to exclude contribution of medications, particularly efavirenz, ZDV, corticosteroids.
2. **Treatment.** SSRI's or tricyclic antidepressants are the mainstays of therapy, as for HIV-negative patients. In general, start with low-doses of all agents and titrate up as needed. Always check treatment guidelines for potential drug interactions with antiretroviral agents (www.aidsinfo.nih.gov). If rapid onset of response is needed, stimulants such as methylphenidate or dextroamphetamine may be tried. MAO inhibitors are contraindicated due to drug interactions.

B. Mania. HIV may produce an unusual form of mania as a manifestation of HIV encephalopathy.

1. **Presentation.** These patients usually have CD4 cell counts < $200/mm^3$. It is distinguished from non-HIV-related bipolar disease in that there is no family history of bipolar illness and onset may occur at any age. Symptoms include expansive mood, grandiosity, and diminished sleep.
2. **Treatment.** Treatment should be undertaken with the assistance of a psychiatrist. Options include lithium 300 mg (PO) q8h or valproic acid 250 mg (PO) q12h or carbamazepine 200 mg (PO) q12h.

C. Insomnia

1. **Etiology.** Sleep disturbance may be a symptom of an underlying medical condition (hepatic encephalopathy, HIV dementia), a psychiatric illness (depression, mania, substance abuse, anxiety), or a medication side effect (efavirenz, corticosteroids).
2. **Treatment.** Attempt to identify/treat underlying causes, including "poor

sleep hygiene" (excessive caffeine, alcohol, other stimulants). For patients with a history of substance abuse, avoid if possible the chronic use of benzodiazepines, which have addictive potential. As an alternative, trazodone 50-100 mg (PO) at bedtime can be very effective. Short-term insomnia due to anxiety or jet lag can be treated with benzodiazepines such as zolpidem (Ambien) 2.5-5.0 mg (PO) at bedtime or lorazepam 1.0 mg (PO) at bedtime.

DERMATOLOGIC COMPLICATIONS

A. Viral Infections

1. **Herpes Simplex Infection.** Oral/anogenital diseases occur more frequently and are more severe in patients with HIV. Infection may also occur on non-mucosal surfaces (e.g., skin), especially when the patient is severely immunocompromised.
   a. **Diagnosis.** Characteristic vesicles on an erythematous base. Ulcerations may occur in primary disease and more advanced HIV-related immunosuppression. A viral culture for HSV is the diagnostic test of choice and is quite sensitive, especially early during the outbreak and prior to starting anti-herpes therapy.
   b. **Treatment.** See p. 84.

2. **Varicella-Zoster Infection.** Herpes zoster is much more common (20-50–fold increased risk) in HIV patients than in age-matched HIV-negative controls and may be first sign of underlying HIV infection. AIDS patients are at increased risk for chronic non-healing zoster, with can last for several weeks. Appearance may also be atypical, with nodular rather than vesicular lesions.
   a. **Diagnosis.** Diagnosed by clinical appearance. DFA test of a lesion can help distinguish zoster from HSV if the diagnosis is unclear.
   b. **Treatment.** See p. 91.

3. **Molluscum Contagiosum**
   a. **Presentation**. Manifests as clusters of white, umbilicated papules outside the groin/perineal area. Rarely seen except with severe immunosuppression (CD4 < 100/mm^3); the number/size of lesions increase as immunosuppression progresses.
   b. **Diagnosis.** Diagnosed by clinical appearance. Biopsy is rarely necessary, but when performed shows large inclusions known as "molluscum bodies." Etiologic virus (a pox virus) cannot be cultured in clinical practice.
   c. **Treatment.** Effective antiretroviral therapy can often lead to dramatic, spontaneous improvement. If this is not possible, or for more immediate control, local cryosurgery or other ablative methods can be effective.

4. **Oral Hairy Leukoplakia (OHL).** See p. 116.

5. **Warts.** Cutaneous and genital warts are extremely common in HIV disease, and in severe cases are disfiguring and difficult to treat. Although usually more severe with progressive HIV disease, in some patients they remain a debilitating problem even with good response to antiretroviral therapy.
   a. **Diagnosis.** Generally a clinical diagnosis. In severe or refractory cases, biopsy is sometimes needed to exclude underlying squamous cell carcinoma.
   b. **Treatment**
      1. **Genital warts.** Imiquimod 5% cream 3x/week at bedtime, wash off in AM. Alternative: podofilox q12h application with cotton swab for 3 days followed by 4 days without treatment, then repeat. Local inflammation is common with both measures. Provider-applied therapies include cryotherapy, podophyllin resin (severe or bulky cases).
      2. **Cutaneous warts.** As in HIV-negative patients, spontaneous resolution may occur, especially in relatively immunocompetent patients. Therapy is otherwise similar as in HIV-negative patients, with multiple ablative therapies available (cryotherapy, liquid nitrogen, salicylic acid, bichloracetic acid, curettage). Refractory cases should be referred to a dermatologist for intra-lesional therapy or wide excision.

B. **Bacterial Infections**
   1. **Staphylococcal Infections.** May cause staphylococcal folliculitis, a pruritic condition associated with small papules. Larger collections of soft tissue staph infection can cause furunculosis or subcutaneous abscesses (more common with advanced HIV-related immunosuppression.) A particular concern has been community MRSA-related soft tissue infections, which are now extremely common in the US, particularly among gay men.
      a. **Diagnosis.** Clinical appearance. Culture to exclude MRSA.
      b. **Treatment.** Dicloxacillin 500 mg (PO) q6h or cephalexin 500 mg (PO) q6h or azithromycin 500 mg (PO) q24h or doxycycline 100 mg (PO) q12h x 7-14 days or until folliculitis resolves. For furunculosis, which is usually due to MRSA, treat according to sensitivities; doxycycline or TMP-SMX 1 DS (PO) q12h are often effective; linezolid 600 mg (PO) q12h is recommended for severe cases. Good local hygiene is also important (keep cuts/abrasions clean with soap and water; launder all bedclothes/towels). For recurrences, consider topical mupirocin ointment to nares q12h x 7 days. Large furuncles or soft tissue collections may need surgical drainage.
   2. **Bacillary Angiomatosis.** A cutaneous manifestation of *Bartonella quintanna* and *Bartonella henselae* infection (cat scratch bacillus); Presents as a dome-shaped and often pedunculated papule or papules in a patient with severe

immunosuppression. Appearance can mimic Kaposi's sarcoma. Organism can also cause hepatic disease (peliosis hepatitis), fever, encephalopathy, endocarditis.

a. **Diagnosis.** Characteristic appearance and biopsy, with pathology showing the characteristic bacillus on Warthin-Starry and Dieterle stains. Organism can be cultured, but laboratory needs to be alerted so special media can be used. Serologies also may be helpful.

b. **Treatment.** Azithromycin 250-500 mg (PO) q24h or clarithromycin 500 mg (PO) q12h or doxycycline 100 mg (PO) q12h. Treatment duration is determined by recovery of immune system in response to antiretroviral therapy.

3. **Syphilis.** See p. 89.

C. Fungal Infections

1. **Disseminated and Invasive Fungal Infections.** All disseminated fungal infections can cause skin lesions. Most characteristic are molluscum-like lesions with cryptococcal disease, erythema nodosum with coccidioides, and nodular skin lesions with blastomycosis.

2. **Tinea Corporis, Cruris, or Pedis (jock itch, athlete's foot).** Extensive erythematous plaques with severe pruritus.

   a. **Diagnosis.** Characteristic appearance, with KOH slide preparation showing branched, septated hyphae.

   b. **Treatment.** Topical therapy with over-the-counter preparations, or by prescription with one of several topical antifungals, including clotrimazole, ciclopirox, or butenafine q12h. For severe disease, use fluconazole 100-200 mg (PO) q24h x 7-14 days or terbinafine 250 mg (PO) q24h x 14 days.

3. **Candidiasis.** In addition to mucosal infections, candida can cause disease in the skin and nails. In the skin, it is often seen in intertriginous areas (groin, under breasts), where it causes a pruritic papular eruption that can coalesce to form large plaques. Web spaces of the fingers and toes may also be involved. Heat and moisture in these areas encourage candidal growth.

   a. **Diagnosis.** Clinically suspected with papular, sometimes pustular eruption in intertriginous areas. A KOH slide shows yeast and pseudohyphae of candida.

   b. **Treatment.** Topical therapy with antifungals, such as clotrimazole q12h x 14 days. More severe cases may require systemic therapy with fluconazole 100-200 mg (PO) q24h x 7-14 days. It is also important to maintain good hygiene, attempt to aerate and dry involved areas, and avoid tight clothing.

D. Miscellaneous Skin Conditions. All can be the first sign of underlying HIV infection.

1. **Seborrheic Dermatitis.** Presents as waxy erythematous and sometimes flakey plaques with scale, usually on face and scalp. Usually worsens with progressive immunodeficiency. May be caused by the yeast *Pityrosporum ovale*. Antiretroviral therapy usually leads to improvement. Symptomatic treatment consists of ketoconazole cream q12h x 7-14 days or a low-potency topical steroid (e.g., hydrocortisone cream 2.5% q12h x 7-14 days). For refractory cases where higher-potency steroids may be indicated, referral to a dermatologist is recommended.
2. **Psoriasis.** Severity of psoriasis correlates with the degree of immunosuppression. HIV can sometimes unmask a prior history of mild disease. May be accompanied by arthritis. Antiretroviral therapy is often useful. Other treatments as per HIV-negative patients.
3. **Eosinophilic Folliculitis.** An erythematous, papular, severely pruritic eruption, usually on the upper trunk and face. Appearance is similar to bacterial folliculitis, but the rash is unresponsive to antibacterials and biopsy demonstrates an eosinophilic infiltrate. The process becomes more difficult to treat as HIV disease progresses; rubbing/scratching can lead to ulcerations, prurigo nodularis, secondary staph infections. In darker-skinned individuals, this can ultimately lead to disfiguring post-inflammatory hyperpigmentation.
   a. **Diagnosis.** Skin biopsy is required.
   b. **Treatment.** The disease is characterized by its refractory nature and frequent relapses. Individual treatments may work well in some individuals but not in others. Options include ART, oral/topical corticosteroids, isotretinoin, and phototherapy. Antiretroviral therapy will ultimately lead to improvement in most patients. However, some individuals go through a paradoxical worsening due to a heightened inflammatory response, which can be difficult to distinguish from an adverse drug reaction and can sometimes last for weeks to months. Prednisone 70 mg (PO) q24h, tapered by 5-10 mg/d, is also helpful. Intermittent therapy of 60 mg (PO) q24h x 2-3 days may be useful to control flares after discontinuation. Potent topical corticosteroids q12h-q8h x 10-14 days can be effective but should not be used on the face. Isotretinoin (Accutane) 1 mg/kg/d or 40 mg (PO) q12h is also of value, with duration determined by response to therapy (associated with skin dryness). Ultraviolet B phototherapy may be used 3x/week until improvement, then maintenance as needed.
4. **Xerosis/Ichthyosis.** Manifests as dry, flakey, and extremely pruritic skin. Worsens as HIV disease progresses, and exacerbated by some antiretrovirals, particularly indinavir. Treatment consists of antiretroviral therapy (avoid indinavir) and emollients (e.g., Aquaphor, Eucerin, Cetaphil). Short-duration (7-14 days) topical steroids may also be considered for dry/inflamed skin.

Chapter 7
HIV Infection and Pregnancy
Ruth Tuomala, MD

HIV AND PREGNANCY

Antiretroviral therapy reduces the risk of perinatal transmission by lowering maternal HIV RNA and by providing pre- and post-exposure prophylaxis for the infant. The Pediatric AIDS Clinical Trials Group (PACTG) Protocol 076 demonstrated a 70% reduction in transmission using single-therapy ZDV. Combination antepartum regimens are even more effective than single-drug regimens and are in concordance with standard-of-care treatment for HIV infection in the non-pregnancy setting. Although the risk of vertical transmission correlates with maternal viral load, there is no maternal viral load below which the risk of transmission is zero. As a result, combination therapy is indicated for all pregnant women, regardless of baseline HIV RNA or CD4 cell count.

INITIAL EVALUATION

Initial evaluation of the HIV-infected pregnant woman requires assessment of the considerations shown in Table 7.1.

Table 7.1. Initial Evaluation of HIV-Infected Pregnant Women

- Degree of immunodeficiency (defined by current and past CD4 cell counts)
- Risk for disease progression and perinatal transmission (determined by HIV RNA)
- If HIV RNA is detectable, whether a resistance genotype is present (determined by resistance testing; previous tests should also be reviewed)
- Need for opportunistic infection prophylaxis
- Baseline hematologic, metabolic, renal, and hepatic parameters
- Complete history of past and current antiretroviral therapy regimens
- Presence of co-infections that might require treatment or special care of the newborn (syphilis, gonorrhea/chlamydia, hepatitis B surface antigen, hepatitis C antibody)
- Assessment of supportive care needs

INITIATION OF ANTIRETROVIRAL THERAPY IN PREGNANCY

Decisions regarding when to start treatment and what regimen to use depends on several factors, including; (1) gestational age of the pregnancy; (2) results of the laboratory testing (Table 7.2); and (3) known, suspected, or unknown effects of individual drugs on the fetus and newborn. An overview of antiretroviral therapy in pregnancy is shown in Tables 7.3 and 7.4.

HIV-infected women in their first trimester of pregnancy who are not on antiretroviral therapy may consider delaying initiation of treatment until after 10-12 weeks gestation, unless they require therapy for their own health, in which case treatment should be started as soon as indicated. For pregnant women with acute HIV infection, treatment should be started immediately given the high HIV RNA levels associated with this condition. Before starting treatment, it is important to emphasize the need for adherence to medical therapy. Patients should also be instructed to have a low threshold for reporting any potential side effects early, especially those that may reduce medication compliance, so that treatment can be altered and/or symptomatic relief for the side effect can be provided.

GOALS OF THERAPY AND MONITORING

The goal of treatment is the same as for non-pregnant individuals: to ensure an undetectable HIV RNA (< 50-75 copies/mL) using the most sensitive available assay. Once antiretroviral therapy is initiated, monitoring of HIV RNA is recommended at 1-2 weeks, then monthly thereafter until the HIV RNA is undetectable, then every 2 months after that. The CD4 cell count should be obtained every 3 months as for non-pregnant adults. Laboratory monitoring for toxicity can be performed at the same time as HIV RNA testing. A general overview of antiretroviral therapy during pregnancy and labor and to the newborn is summarized in Table 7.2.

In the case of virologic failure — i.e., inability to achieve an undetectable HIV RNA or viral rebound occurs — repeat resistance testing is indicated. Subsequent management will depend on assessment of medication adherence and the degree of resistance detected on testing, as described in Chapter 4. For women who have not achieved virologic suppression near the time of delivery, especially if the HIV RNA exceeds 1000 copies/mL, a scheduled cesarean delivery is recommended at 38 weeks gestation.

Table 7.2. Overview of Antiretroviral Therapy (ART) During Pregnancy, Labor, and to the Infant Post-Partum

Setting	Regimen
Antepartum	Combination ART should be started with a goal of HIV RNA suppression. Women who require ART solely to prevent perinatal HIV transmission may wish to delay starting therapy until after week 10-12 of gestation. If treatment is needed for maternal health based on standard adult treatment guidelines, it should be started when indicated, even during the first trimester. ZDV should be included in the regimen unless there is severe toxicity or resistance. Commonly used regimens include ZDV/3TC (co-formulated) plus a boosted PI such as LPV/r, ATV/r, or SQV/r. EFV should not be used (especially in the first trimester) due to animal data showing increased risk of CNS defects, and NFV should not be used because it contains ethyl methane sulfonate (EMS), a potential teratogen. Nevirapine may be considered only if the maternal CD4 cell count is < 250 cells/mm^3
Intrapartum	ZDV is administered intravenously, with a loading dose of 2 mg/kg over 1 hour, followed by continuous infusion of 1 mg/kg/hr until delivery. Other components of the antiretroviral regimen are continued through delivery, with the exception of d4T (potential antagonism between ZDV and d4T)
Postpartum	Combination ART is continued if indicated based on maternal clinical and immunological status. Women taking ART solely to prevent vertical transmission may elect to discontinue therapy at this time. Infants should receive oral ZDV syrup at a dose of 2 mg/kg q6h for the first 6 weeks of life. Infants born to women with known ZDV resistance should have their post-partum regimen selected in consultation with a pediatric Infectious Diseases/HIV specialist

MANAGEMENT OF HIV-INFECTED PREGNANT WOMEN CURRENTLY RECEIVING ANTIRETROVIRAL THERAPY

Women currently receiving a suppressive antiretroviral regimen at the onset of pregnancy should continue the successful regimen, even in the first trimester. Discontinuation of therapy will lead to virologic rebound, potentially increasing the risk of disease progression, viral resistance, and vertical transmission. In general, the same suppressive regimen should be continued unless the regimen includes

EFV or NFV. EFV should be avoided during pregnancy (especially in the first trimester), and NFV is no longer recommended during pregnancy since it contains ethyl methane sulfonate (EMS), a process-related impurity shown in animal studies to be teratogenic, mutagenic, and carcinogenic. Although no excess risk of birth defects has been reported yet in infants born to pregnant women who have received NFV, pregnant women should not be offered regimens containing this drug until further notice. Similarly, women who are trying to conceive or who are sexually active without using effective or consistent contraception should not receive EFV- or NFV-containing regimens.

Women receiving a non-suppressive antiretroviral regimen at the onset of pregnancy should undergo assessment for virologic failure as described in Chapter 3. Selection of the optimal regimen is based on medication adherence, results of resistance testing, and understanding the known and unknown safety issues associated with antiretroviral agents in pregnancy.

In general, if antiretroviral therapy is given solely for prevention of perinatal HIV transmission, the regimen may be discontinued after delivery with a low risk of HIV disease progression in the mother. Depending on the pre-treatment CD4 cell count and tolerability of the regimen, some women may elect to continue treatment given the possible benefits of early therapy and hence should be given this option. During pregnancy, if treatment must be stopped for severe toxicity or pregnancy-induced hyperemesis, all drugs should generally be stopped at the same time and then reinitiated together. The exception to this practice is for NNRTI-based treatment; if possible, the NRTI backbone should be continued for 7 days after stopping the NRTI to avoid selecting for NNRTI resistance.

OTHER MANAGEMENT AND MONITORING MEASURES

A. Other Management Considerations. Pregnant HIV-infected women should be instructed to discontinue cigarettes, illicit drugs and unprotected sex, and to avoid breastfeeding. Prophylaxis against opportunistic infections is indicated as for nonpregnant HIV-infected women (Chapter 5). Because of concern over antiretroviral therapy and an increase in pregnancy-induced hyperglycemia, standard glucose-loading tests should be performed earlier in pregnancy than typical, and then repeated in the third trimester.

B. Fetal Monitoring. Specific adverse obstetrical outcomes have not been ascribed to antiretroviral therapy. Nevertheless, many providers monitor fetal anatomy, growth, and well-being with regular frequency using ultrasound, non-stress testing, and biophysical profiles. Specifically, first trimester ultrasound is recommended to confirm gestational age and to guide the timing of scheduled cesarean delivery (recommended at 38 weeks gestation for women who have not achieved virologic suppression). For patients not seen until later in gestation, second trimester ultrasound can be used to assess fetal anatomy and determine gestational age. Second trimester ultrasound assessment of fetal anatomy is also recommended for women receiving combination antiretroviral therapy during the first trimester, especially if the regimen included EFV. Third trimester ultrasound assessment of fetal growth and well-being should also be considered for woman receiving a combination drug regimen for which there is limited experience with use in pregnancy. The need for non-stress testing and other assessments is based on ultrasound findings and the presence of maternal comorbidities.

POSTPARTUM MANAGEMENT

Children born to HIV-infected women need to be assessed for the possibility of HIV infection and for short- and long-term toxicities due to in-utero exposure to antiretroviral agents. Exposure to antiretroviral agents should become a part of the child's permanent medical record. Further arrangements are needed for long-term care of the woman, including primary and HIV-specialty care appointments, made prior to hospital discharge, and family planning counseling. Mental health status and the possibility of postpartum depression also need to be assessed, and appropriate supports need to be put into place. The importance of adherence to antiretroviral therapy postpartum should be stressed at every patient visit. Case management services best assure adequate support and compliance with health care needs.

Table 7.3. Antiretroviral Drug Classes Used in Pregnant HIV-Infected Women (also see Table 7.4 for information on individual drugs)

Drug Class	Concerns in Pregnancy	Use in Pregnancy
NRTI's	Potential maternal and infant mitochondrial toxicity	NRTI's are recommended for use as part of combination regimens, usually including 2 NRTI's with either an NNRTI or one or more PI's. Use of single or dual NRTI's alone is not recommended for treatment of HIV infection (ZDV alone may be considered for prophylaxis of perinatal transmission in pregnant women with HIV RNA < 1,000 copies/mL)
NNRTI's	Hypersensitivity reactions, including hepatic toxicity and rash, more common in women; unclear if increased in pregnancy	NNRTI's are recommended for use in combination regimens with 2 NRTI drugs
Protease Inhibitors (PI's)	Hyperglycemia, new onset or exacerbation of diabetes mellitus, and diabetic ketoacidosis reported with PI use; unclear if pregnancy increases risk. Conflicting data regarding preterm delivery in women receiving PI's	PI's are recommended for use in combination regimens with 2 NRTI drugs
Entry Inhibitors (fusion inhibitors, CCR5 antagonists)	Minimal data in human pregnancy	Safety and pharmacokinetics data in pregnancy are insufficient to recommend use during pregnancy
Integrase Inhibitors	No experience in human pregnancy	Safety and pharmacokinetics data in pregnancy are insufficient to recommend use during pregnancy

From: Public Health Service Recommendation for Use of Antiretroviral Drugs in Pregnant HIV-Infected Women for Maternal Health and Interventions to Reduce Perinatal HIV Transmission in the United States. November 2, 2007. www.hivatis.org.

Table 7.4. Antiretroviral Drug Used in Pregnant HIV-Infected Woman (also see Table 7.3 for information on drug classes)

NUCLEOSIDE (AND NUCLEOTIDE) REVERSE TRANSCRIPTASE INHIBITORS (NRTI'S)		
Recommended agents	Zidovudine*	Preferred NRTI for use in combination ART in pregnancy based on efficacy studies and extensive experience; should be included in regimen unless significant toxicity or stavudine use. No evidence of human teratogenicity. Well-tolerated, short-term safety demonstrated for mother and infant. No change in dose during pregnancy is required
	Lamivudine*	Because of extensive experience with lamivudine in pregnancy in combination with zidovudine, lamivudine plus zidovudine is the recommended dual NRTI backbone for pregnant women. No evidence of human teratogenicity. Well-tolerated, short-term safety demonstrated for mother and infant. No change in dose during pregnancy is required
Alternate agents	Didanosine	Alternate NRTI for dual nucleoside backbone of combination regimens. Didanosine should be used with stavudine only if no other alternatives are available. Cases of lactic acidosis, some fatal, have been reported in pregnant women receiving didanosine and stavudine together. No change in dose during pregnancy is required
	Emtricitabine†	Alternate NRTI for dual nucleoside backbone of combination regimens. No studies in human pregnancy is required
	Stavudine	Alternate NRTI for dual nucleoside backbone of combination regimens. Stavudine should be used with didanosine only if no other alternatives are available. Do not use with zidovudine due to potential for antagonism. No evidence of human teratogenicity. Cases of lactic acidosis, some fatal, have been reported in pregnant women receiving didanosine and stavudine together. No change in dose during pregnancy is required
	Abacavir*	Alternate NRTI for dual nucleoside backbone of combination regimens. See footnote regarding use in triple NRTI regimen.# Hypersensitivity reactions occur in ~5%-8% of nonpregnant persons; a much smaller percentage are fatal and are usually associated with rechallenge. Rate in pregnancy unknown. Educate patient regarding symptoms of hypersensitivity. No change in dose during pregnancy is required. Only use if HLA-B*5701 negative

Table 7.4. Antiretroviral Drug Used in Pregnant HIV-Infected Woman (also see Table 7.3 for information on drug classes) (cont'd)

NUCLEOSIDE (AND NUCLEOTIDE) REVERSE TRANSCRIPTASE INHIBITORS (NRTI'S)		
Insufficient data to recommend use	Tenofovir†	Because of lack of data on use in human pregnancy and concern regarding potential fetal bone effects, tenofovir should be used as a component of a maternal combination regimen only after careful consideration of alternatives. Studies in monkeys show decreased fetal growth and reduction in fetal bone porosity within 2 months of starting maternal therapy
Not recommended	Zalcitabine (no longer available in the United States)	Given lack of data and concerns regarding teratogenicity in animals, not recommended for use in human pregnancy unless alternatives are not available
NON-NUCLEOSIDE REVERSE TRANSCRIPTASE INHIBITORS (NNRTI'S)		
Recommended agents	Nevirapine	Nevirapine should be initiated in pregnant women with CD4 counts > 250 cells/mm3 only if benefit clearly outweighs risk, due to the increased risk of potentially life-threatening hepatotoxicity in women with high CD4 counts. Women who enter pregnancy on nevirapine regimens and are tolerating them well may continue therapy, regardless of CD4 count. No evidence of human teratogenicity. No change in dose during pregnancy is required
Not recommended	Efavirenz†	Use of efavirenz should be avoided in the first trimester, and women of childbearing potential must be counseled regarding risks and avoidance of pregnancy. Because of the known failure rates of contraception, alternate regimens should be strongly considered in women of child-bearing potential. Use after the second trimester of pregnancy can be considered if other alternatives are not available and if adequate contraception can be assured postpartum. FDA Pregnancy Class D
	Delavirdine	Given lack of data and concerns about teratogenicity in animals, not recommended for use in human pregnancy unless alternatives are unavailable

Table 7.4. Antiretroviral Drug Used in Pregnant HIV-Infected Woman (also see Table 7.3 for information on drug classes) (cont'd)

PROTEASE INHIBITORS (PI'S)		
Recommended agents	Lopinavir/ritonavir	The capsule formulation is no longer available. Pharmacokinetic studies of the new tablet formulation are underway, but there are currently insufficient data to make a definitive recommendation regarding dosing in pregnancy. Some experts would administer standard dosing (2 tablets twice daily) throughout pregnancy and monitor virologic response and lopinavir drug levels, if available. Other experts, extrapolating from the capsule formulation pharmacokinetic data, would increase the dose of the tablet formulation during the third trimester (from 2 tablets to 3 tablets twice daily), returning to standard dosing postpartum. Once daily lopinavir/ritonavir dosing is not recommended during pregnancy (no data to address whether drug levels are adequate). No evidence of human teratogenicity. Well-tolerated, short-term safety demonstrated in Phase I/II studies
Alternate agents	Indinavir	Alternate PI to consider if unable to use lopinavir/ritonavir, but would need to give indinavir as ritonavir-boosted regimen. Optimal dosing for the combination of indinavir/ritonavir in pregnancy is unknown. Theoretical concern re: increased indirect bilirubin levels, which may exacerbate physiologic hyperbilirubinemia in the neonate, but minimal placental passage. Use of unboosted indinavir during pregnancy is not recommended
	Ritonavir	Given low levels in pregnant women when used alone, recommended for use in combination with second PI as low-dose ritonavir "boost" to increase levels of second PI
	Saquinavir-hard gel capsule [HGC] (Invirase)/ritonavir	There are limited pharmacokinetic data on saquinavir-HGC and the new tablet formulation in pregnancy. Ritonavir-boosted saquinavir-HGC or saquinavir tablets are alternative PI's for combination regimens in pregnancy, and are alternative initial antiretroviral recommendations for non-pregnant adults. Well-tolerated, short-term safety demonstrated for mother and infant for both saquinavir-SGC and -HGC in combination with low-dose ritonavir. Limited pharmacokinetic data on saquinavir-HGC, and the new 500-mg tablet formulation, suggest that 1,000 mg saquinavir-HGC/100 mg ritonavir given twice daily achieves adequate saquinavir drug levels in pregnant women

Table 7.4. Antiretroviral Drug Used in Pregnant HIV-Infected Woman (also see Table 7.3 for information on drug classes) (cont'd)

	PROTEASE INHIBITORS (PI'S)	
Insufficient data to recommend use	Amprenavir, atazanavir, darunavir, fosamprenavir, tipranavir	Safety and pharmacokinetics data in pregnancy are insufficient to recommend use during pregnancy. Clinical trials of ATV/r in pregnancy are ongoing
Not recommended	Nelfinavir	Not currently recommended for use in pregnancy until further notice unless no alternative is available. In September 2007, the manufacturer sent a letter to providers regarding the presence of low levels of ethyl methane sulfonate (EMS), a process-related impurity, in nelfinavir. EMS is teratogenic, mutagenic and carcinogenic in animals, although no data from humans exist and no increase in birth defects has been observed in the Antiretroviral Pregnancy Registry
	ENTRY INHIBITORS	
Insufficient data to recommend use	Enfuvirtide (fusion inhibitor), maraviroc (CCR5 antagonist)	Safety and pharmacokinetics data in pregnancy are insufficient to recommend use during pregnancy
	INTEGRASE INHIBITORS	
Insufficient data to recommend use	Raltegravir	Safety and pharmacokinetics data in pregnancy are insufficient to recommend use during pregnancy

HCG = hard gel capsule; NRTI = nucleoside reverse transcriptase inhibitor; NtRTI = nucleotide reverse transcriptase inhibitor; NNRTI = non-nucleoside reverse transcriptase inhibitor; PI = protease inhibitor; SGC = soft gel capsule.

* Zidovudine and lamivudine are included as a fixed-dose combination in Combivir; zidovudine, lamivudine, and abacavir are included as a fixed-dose combination in Trizivir.

† Emtricitabine and tenofovir are included as a fixed-dose combination in Truvada; emtricitabine, tenofovir, and efavirenz are included as a fixed-dose combination in Atripla.

Triple NRTI regimens including abacavir have been less potent virologicaly compared to PI-based regimens. Triple NRTI regimens should be used only when an NNRTI- or PI-based regimen cannot be used (e.g., due to significant drug interactions). A study evaluating use of zidovudine/lamivudine/abacavir among pregnant women with HIV RNA < 55,000 copies/mL as a class-a sparing regimen is in development.

From: Public Health Service Recommendation for Use of Antiretroviral Drugs in Pregnant HIV-Infected Women for Maternal Health and Interventions to Reduce Perinatal HIV Transmission in the United States. November 2, 2007. www.hivatis.org.

Chapter 8
Post-Exposure Prophylaxis

OCCUPATIONAL POST-EXPOSURE PROPHYLAXIS (PEP)

The CDC estimates > 600,000 significant exposures to blood-borne pathogens occur yearly. Of 56 confirmed cases of HIV acquisition in healthcare workers, more than 90% involved percutaneous exposure, with the remaining cases due to mucous membrane/non-intact skin exposure. Estimates of HIV seroconversion rates after percutaneous and mucous membrane exposure to HIV-infected blood are 0.3% and 0.09%, respectively; lower rates of transmission occur after nonintact skin exposure, and no transmission has thus far been reported to occur through intact skin. (By comparison, the risks of seroconversion after percutaneous exposure to Hepatitis B and Hepatitis C viruses are 30% and 3%, respectively.) Risk factors for increased risk of HIV transmission after percutaneous exposure include deep injury (odds ratio 16.1), visible blood on device (odds ratio 5.2), source patient is terminally ill (odds ratio 6.4), or needle was in source patient's artery/vein (odds ratio 5.1); ZDV prophylaxis reduces the risk of transmission (OR 0.2). All guidelines suggest PEP should be administered as soon as possible after exposure, but there is no absolute window (e.g., within 1-2 weeks) after which PEP should be withheld following serious exposure. Because clear-cut efficacy data for patient selection and PEP regimens are lacking, most experts rely on CDC guidelines, which emphasize the type of exposure and potential infectivity of the source patient (Tables 8.1, 8.2). The latest U.S. Public Health Service (USPHS) guidelines for the management of occupational exposure to HIV and postexposure prophylaxis are summarized below and are detailed in Morbidity Mortality Weekly Review 54(RR9):1-17, Sept 30, 2005, or at www.aidsinfo.nih.gov/guidelines. Additional information can be found at the National Clinicians' Postexposure Prophylaxis Hotline (www.ucsf.edu/hivcntr). Occupationally acquired HIV infections and PEP failures should be reported to the CDC at (800) 893-0485.

Recommendations from the updated 2005 USPHS guidelines include:

- Initiate PEP as soon as possible after exposure (preferably within hours), and continue PEP for 4 weeks if tolerated (Tables 8.1, 8.2)
- Seek expert consultation if viral resistance is suspected
- Offer pregnancy testing to all women of childbearing age not known to be pregnant
- Advise exposed persons to seek medical evaluation for any acute illness during follow-up
- Perform HIV-antibody testing and HIV RNA testing for any illness compatible with an acute retroviral syndrome (e.g., pharyngitis, fever, rash, myalgia, fatigue, malaise, lymphadenopathy)
- Perform HIV-antibody testing for at least 6 months postexposure (at baseline, 6 weeks, 3 months, and 6 months)
- Advise exposed persons to use precautions to prevent secondary transmission during follow-up, especially during the first 6-12 weeks, when most HIV-infected patients will seroconvert. Precautions include sexual abstinence or use of condoms, refrain from donating blood, plasma, organs, tissue or semen, and discontinuation of breast-feeding after high-risk exposures
- Evaluate exposed persons taking PEP within 72 hours after exposure, and monitor for drug toxicity for at least 2 weeks. Approximately 50% will experience nausea, malaise, headache, or anorexia, and about one-third will discontinue PEP due to drug toxicity. Lab monitoring should include (at a minimum) a CBC, serum creatinine, liver function tests, serum glucose (if receiving a protease inhibitor to detect hyperglycemia), and monitoring for HBV and HCV. Serious adverse events should be reported to the FDA's MedWatch Program
- If available, employees with workplace exposure should follow up in their designated occupational health sites according to employer policies. This will help retain rights and/or benefits defined by the job in case of infection

Table 8.1. Recommendations for Occupation HIV Postexposure Prophylaxis (see Table 8.2 for basic and expanded PEP regimens)

Exposure Type	Infection Status of Source Patient				
	HIV (+) Class 1*	HIV (+) Class 2*	HIV status unknown[†]	Unknown source[††]	HIV (–)
Percutaneous injuries *Less severe*[+]	Recommend basic 2-drug PEP	Recommend expanded 3-drug PEP	Generally no PEP warranted; consider basic 2-drug PEP[†††] for source with HIV risk factors**	Generally no PEP warranted; consider basic 2-drug PEP[†††] if exposure to HIV-infected persons is likely	No PEP warranted
More severe[+]	Recommend expanded 3-drug PEP	Recommend expanded ≥ 3-drug PEP			
Mucous membrane/ nonintact skin exposure *Small volume*[++]	Consider basic 2-drug PEP	Recommend basic 2-drug PEP			
Large volume[++]	Recommend basic 2-drug PEP	Recommend expanded ≥ 3-drug PEP			

HIV (+) = HIV-positive, HIV (–) = HIV-negative, PEP = postexposure prophylaxis

* Class 1: Asymptomatic HIV infection or known low HIV RNA (e.g., < 1500 RNA copies/mL) Class 2: Symptomatic HIV infection, AIDS, acute seroconversion, or known high HIV RNA. If drug resistance is a concern, obtain expert consultation; do not delay PEP pending consultation

** Source with HIV risk factors: If PEP is administered and the source patient is later determined to be HIV-negative, PEP should be discontinued

† HIV status unknown: for example, source patient is deceased with no samples available for HIV testing

†† Unknown source: for example, a needle from a sharps disposal container (percutaneous injury)

††† PEP is optional; discuss with patient and individualize decision

\+ Less severe: for example, a solid needle and superficial injury. More severe: for example, a large-bore hollow needle, deep puncture, visible blood on device, or needle used in patient's artery/vein

++ Small volume: a few drops. Large volume: major blood splash

From: Updated U.S. Public Health Service Guidelines for the Management of Occupational Exposures to HBV, HCV, and HIV and Recommendations for Postexposure Prophylaxis, MMWR, 50 (RR-9):1-17, September 30, 2005 (www.aidsinfo.nih.gov)

Table 8.2. Basic and Expanded Occupational HIV Postexposure Prophylaxis Regimens (see Table 8.1 for patient selection guidelines)

Regimen	Dosage	Comments
Basic regimen *Preferred*	Zidovudine 300 mg bid or 200 mg tid with food + lamivudine 300 mg qd or 150 mg bid. Available as Combivir tablet: dose = 1 tablet bid	Advantages: ZDV associated with decreased risk for HIV transmission; ZDV used more often than other drugs for PEP for health-care personnel (HCP); serious toxicity rare when used for PEP; side effects predictable and manageable with antimotility and antiemetic agents; can be used by pregnant HCP; can be given as a single tablet (COMBIVIR™) twice daily Disadvantages: side effects (especially nausea and fatigue) common and might result in low adherence; source-patient virus resistance to this regimen possible; potential for delayed toxicity (oncogenic/teratogenic) unknown
	Zidovudine 300 mg bid or 200 mg tid with food + emtricitabine 200 mg (one capsule) qd	Advantages: ZDV: see above; convenient (once daily); well tolerated; long intracellular half-life (~ 40 hours) Disadvantages: ZDV: see above; FTC: rash perhaps more frequent than with 3TC; no long-term experience with this drug; cross resistance to 3TC; hyperpigmentation among non-Caucasians with long-term use: 3%
	Tenofovir 300 mg qd + lamivudine 300 mg qd or 150 mg bid	Advantages: 3TC: see above; TDF: convenient dosing (single pill once daily); resistance profile activity against certain thymidine analogue mutations; well tolerated Disadvantages: TDF: same class warnings as nucleoside reverse transcriptase inhibitors (NRTI's); drug interactions; increased TDF concentrations among persons taking atazanavir and lopinavir/ritonavir; need to monitor patients for TDF-associated toxicities; preferred dosage of atazanavir if used with TDF: ATV 300 mg + ritonavir 100 mg once daily + TDF 300 mg once daily
	Tenofovir 300 mg qd + emtricitabine 200 mg qd. Available as Truvada tablet: dose = 1 tablet qd	Advantages: FTC: see above; TDF: convenient dosing (single pill once daily Truvada); resistance profile activity against certain thymidine analogue mutations; well tolerated Disadvantages: TDF: same class warnings as (NRTI's); drug interactions; increased TDF concentrations among persons taking atazanavir and lopinavir/ritonavir; need to monitor patients for TDF-associated toxicities; preferred dosage of atazanavir if used with TDF: ATV 300 mg + ritonavir 100 mg once daily + TDF 300 mg once daily

Table 8.2. Basic and Expanded Occupational HIV Postexposure Prophylaxis Regimens (see Table 8.1 for patient selection guidelines) (cont'd)

Regimen	Dosage	Comments
Basic regimen *Alternate*	Lamivudine 300 mg qd or 150 mg bid + stavudine 40 mg bid (can use lower doses of 20-30 mg bid if toxicity occurs) or 30 mg bid for body weight < 60 kg	Advantages: 3TC: see above; d4T: gastrointestinal (GI) side effects rare Disadvantages: possibility that source-patient virus is resistant to this regimen; potential for delayed toxicity (oncogenic/teratogenic) unknown
	Emtricitabine 200 mg qd + stavudine 40 mg bid (can use lower doses of 20-30 mg bid if toxicity occurs) or 30 mg bid for body weight < 60 kg	Advantages: 3TC: see above; d4T's GI side effects rare Disadvantages: potential that source-patient virus is resistant to this regimen; unknown potential for delayed toxicity (oncogenic/teratogenic) unknown
Expanded regimen *Preferred*	Basic regimen plus: Lopinavir/ritonavir (Kaletra) 400/100 mg = 2 tablets bid with or without food	Advantages: potent HIV protease inhibitor; generally well-tolerated Disadvantages: potential for serious or life-threatening drug interactions (Chapter 3); might accelerate clearance of certain drugs, including oral contraceptives (requiring alternative or additional contraceptive measures for women taking these drugs); can cause severe hyperlipidemia, especially hypertriglyceridemia; GI (e.g., diarrhea) events common
Alternate (basic regimen plus one of the following drugs)	Atazanavir. 400 mg qd, or atazanavir 300 mg qd + ritonavir 100 mg qd	Advantages: potent HIV protease inhibitor; convenient dosing - once daily; generally well-tolerated Disadvantages: hyperbilirubinemia and jaundice common; potential for serious or life-threatening drug interactions (Chapter 3); avoid coadministration with proton pump inhibitors; separate antacids and buffered medications by 2 hours and H2-receptor antagonists by 12 hours to avoid decreasing ATV levels; caution should be used with ATV and products known to induce PR prolongation (e.g., diltiazem)
	Fosamprenavir 1400 mg bid (without ritonavir), or fosamprenavir 1400 mg qd + ritonavir 200 mg qd, or fosamprenavir 700 mg bid + ritonavir 100 mg bid	Advantages: once daily dosing when given with ritonavir Disadvantages: tolerability: GI side effects common; multiple drug interactions. Oral contraceptives decrease fosamprenavir concentrations; incidence of rash in healthy volunteers, especially when used with low doses of ritonavir. Differentiating between early drug-associated rash and acute seroconversion can be difficult and cause extraordinary concern for the exposed person

Table 8.2. Basic and Expanded Occupational HIV Postexposure Prophylaxis Regimens (see Table 8.1 for patient selection guidelines) (cont'd)

Regimen	Dosage	Comments
Expanded regimen *(cont'd)* *Alternate* *(basic regimen plus one of the following drugs)*	Indinavir 800 mg bid + ritonavir 100 mg bid without regard to food, or indinavir 800 mg tid on empty stomach	Advantages: potent HIV inhibitor Disadvantages: potential for serious or life-threatening drug interactions; serious toxicity (e.g., nephrolithiasis) possible; consumption of 8 glasses of fluid/day required; hyperbilirubinemia common; must avoid this drug during late pregnancy; requires acid for absorption and cannot be taken simultaneously with ddI, chewable/dispersible buffered tablet formulation (doses must be separated by ≥ 1 hour)
	Saquinavir 1000 mg (given as Invirase) bid + ritonavir 100 mg bid	Advantages: generally well-tolerated, although GI events common Disadvantages: potential for serious or life-threatening drug interactions (Chapter 3)
	Nelfinavir 1250 mg (2 x 625-mg tablets or 5 x 250-mg tablets) bid with a meal	Advantages: generally well-tolerated, although diarrhea common Disadvantages: potential for serious or life-threatening drug interactions (Chapter 3); diarrhea
	Efavirenz 600 mg once daily at bedtime	Advantages: does not require phosphorylation before activation and might be active earlier than other antiretroviral agents (a theoretic advantage of no demonstrated clinical benefit); once daily dosing Disadvantages: drug associated with rash (early onset) that can be severe and might rarely progress to Stevens-Johnson syndrome; differentiating between early drug-associated rash and acute seroconversion can be difficult and cause extraordinary concern for the exposed person; CNS side effects (e.g., dizziness, somnolence, insomnia, or abnormal dreaming) common; severe psychiatric symptoms possible (dosing before bedtime might minimize these side effects); teratogen; should not be used during pregnancy; potential for serious or life-threatening drug interactions (Chapter 3)

Adapted from: U.S. Public Health Service Guidelines. MMWR 54(RR-9):1-17, September 30, 2005

NONOCCUPATIONAL POST-EXPOSURE PROPHYLAXIS (nPEP)

In January, 2005, the U.S. Department of Health and Human Services issued recommendations for antiretroviral PEP after sexual, injection-drug use, and other nonoccupational exposures to HIV (MMWR 2005;54(RR-2):1-28).

A. **Evaluation.** The evaluation of person seeking nonoccupational PEP should include determination of the HIV status of the potentially exposed person, the timing and characteristics of the most recent exposure, the frequency of exposures to HIV, the HIV status of the source, and the likelihood of concomitant infection with other pathogens. Available data indicate that nonoccupational PEP is less likely to be effective if initiated > 72 hours after HIV exposure. Therefore, if initiation of nonoccupational PEP is delayed, the likelihood of benefit might not outweigh the risks associated with antiretroviral medications. Persons who engage in behaviors that result in frequent, recurrent exposures that would require sequential or near-continuous courses of antiretroviral medications (e.g., discordant sex partners who rarely use condoms or injection-drug users who often share injection equipment) should not take nonoccupational PEP. In these instances, exposed persons should instead be provided with intensive risk-reduction interventions. If the risk associated with the exposure is considered substantial, nonoccupational PEP can be started pending determination of the HIV status of the source and then stopped if the source is determined to be noninfected. The highest levels of estimated per-act risk for HIV transmission are associated with blood transfusion, needle sharing by injection-drug users, receptive anal intercourse, and percutaneous needlestick injuries. Insertive anal intercourse, penile-vaginal exposures, and oral sex represent substantially less per-act risk.

B. **Use of Antiretroviral Therapy (Table 8.1).** A 28-day course of antiretroviral therapy is recommended for persons who have had nonoccupational exposure to blood, genital secretions, or other potentially infected body fluids of a persons known to be HIV infected when: (1) that exposure represents a substantial risk for HIV transmission (Figure 8.1); and (2) when the person seeks care within 72 hours of exposure. When indicated, antiretroviral nonoccupational PEP should be initiated promptly for the best chance of success. No evidence indicates that a 3-drug regimen is more likely to be effective than a 2-drug regimen. If there is concern about potential adherence and toxicity issues associated with a 3-drug regimen, a 2-drug regimen may be considered (i.e., a combination of two reverse transcriptase inhibitors). When the source-person is available for interview, their history of antiretroviral medication use and most recent viral load measurement might help avoid prescribing antiretroviral medications to which the source-virus is likely to be resistant. If the source-person is willing, it may be useful to draw blood for viral load and resistance testing if the results can be obtained promptly.

C. Follow-up Testing. All patients seeking care after HIV exposure should be tested for the presence of HIV antibodies at baseline and at 4–6 weeks, 3 months, and 6 months after exposure to determine whether HIV infection has occurred. In addition, testing for sexually transmitted diseases, hepatitis B and C, and pregnancy should be offered (Table 8.3). Patients should be instructed about the signs and symptoms associated with acute retroviral infection especially fever and rash, and asked to return for evaluation if these occur during or after nonoccupational PEP.

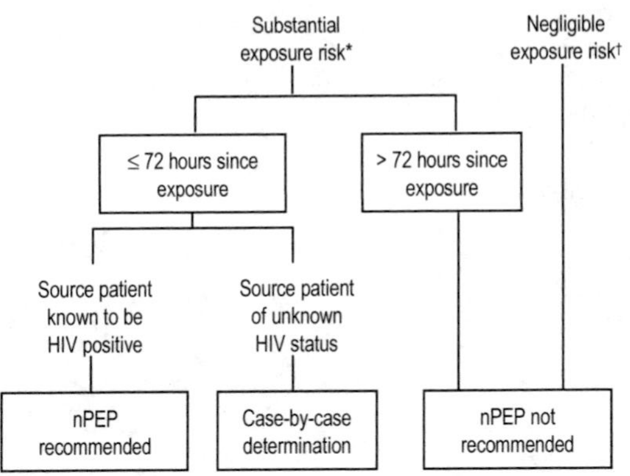

Figure 8.1. Evaluation and Treatment of Possible Nonoccupational HIV Exposures

nPEP = nonoccupational post-exposure prophylaxis

* Substantial risk for HIV exposure = exposure of vagina, rectum, eye, mouth, or other mucous membrane, nonintact skin, or percutaneous contact with blood, semen, vaginal secretions, rectal secretions, breast milk, or any body fluid that is visibly contaminated with blood when the source is know to be HIV-infected

† Negligible risk for HIV exposure = exposure of vagina, rectum, eye, mouth, or other mucous membrane, intact or nonintact skin, or percutaneous contact with urine, nasal secretions, saliva, sweat, or tears if not visibly contaminated with blood regardless of the known or suspected HIV status of the source

Table 8.3. Recommended Laboratory Evaluation for Nonoccupational Postexposure Prophylaxis (nPEP) of HIV Infection

Test	Baseline	During nPEP*	Time After Exposure		
			4-6 Weeks	3 Months	6 Months
HIV antibody testing	E, S		E	E	E
Complete blood count with differential	E	E			
Serum liver enzymes	E	E			
Sexually transmitted diseases screen (gonorrhea, chlamydia, syphilis)	E, S	E¶	E¶		
Hepatitis B serology	E, S		E¶	E¶	
Hepatitis C serology	E, S			E	E
Pregnancy test (women of reproductive age)	E	E¶	E¶		
HIV viral load	S		E**	E**	E**
HIV resistance testing	S		E**	E**	E**
CD4+ T lymphocyte count	S		E**	E**	E**

E = exposed patient, S = source

* Other specific tests might be indicated depending on antiretrovirals prescribed. Literature pertaining to individual agents should be consulted

§ HIV antibody testing of the source patient is indicated for sources of unknown serostatus

¶ Additional testing for pregnancy, sexually transmitted diseases, and hepatitis B should be performed as clinically indicated

** If determined to be HIV infected on follow-up testing; perform as clinically indicated once diagnosed

From: Antiretroviral Postexposure Prophylaxis after Sexual, Injection-drug Use, or Other Nonoccupational Exposure to HIV in the United States. MMWR January 21, 2005, 54 (No. RR-2):1-16

Chapter 9

Antiretroviral Drug Summaries

David W. Kubiak, PharmD, BCPS
Demary Torres, PharmD

This section contains prescribing information pertinent to the clinical use of antiretroviral agents in adults, as compiled from a variety of sources, including MICROMEDEX®, Up to Date on-line version 14.2®, Department of Health and Human Services Guidelines for the use of antiretroviral agents in HIV-1-infected adults and adolescents (www.aidsinfo.nih.gov/guidelines/), January 29, 2008, manufacturers' product information, among others. The information provided is not exhaustive, and the reader is referred to other drug information references and the manufacturer's product literature for further information. Clinical use of the information provided and any consequences that may arise from its use are the responsibilities of the prescribing physician. The authors, editors, and publisher do not warrant or guarantee the information contained in this section, and do not assume and expressly disclaim any liability for errors or omissions or any consequences that may occur from such. **The use of any drug should be preceded by careful review of the package insert, which provides indications and dosing approved by the U.S. Food and Drug Administration. This information can be obtained on the website provided at the end of the reference list for each drug summary.**

Drugs are listed alphabetically by generic name; trade names follow in parentheses. To search by trade name, consult the index. Each drug summary contains the following information:

Usual Dose. Represents the usual dose to treat HIV infection in adult patients with normal hepatic and renal function. Additional information can be found in the manufacturer's package insert and product literature.

Bioavailability. Refers to the percentage of the dose reaching the systemic circulation from the site of administration (PO or IM). For PO antibiotics, bioavailability refers to the percentage of dose adsorbed from the GI tract.

Excreted Unchanged. Refers to the percentage of drug excreted unchanged, and provides an indirect measure of drug concentration in the urine/feces.

Serum Half-Life (normal/ESRD). The serum half-life ($T_{1/2}$) is the time (in hours) in which serum concentration falls by 50%. Serum half-life is useful in determining dosing interval. If the half-life of drugs eliminated by the kidneys is prolonged in end-stage renal disease (ESRD), then the total daily dose is reduced in proportion to the degree of renal dysfunction. If the half-life in ESRD is similar to the normal half-life, then the total daily dose does not change.

Plasma Protein Binding. Expressed as the percentage of drug reversibly bound to serum albumin. It is the unbound (free) portion of a drug that equilibrates with tissues and imparts antiviral activity. Plasma protein binding is not typically a factor in antimicrobial effectiveness unless binding exceeds 95%. Decreases in serum albumin (nephrotic syndrome, liver disease) or competition for protein binding from other drugs or endogenously produced substances (uremia, hyperbilirubinemia) will increase the percentage of free drug available for antimicrobial activity, and may require a decrease in dosage. Increases in serum binding proteins (trauma, surgery, critical illness) will decrease the percentage of free drug available for antimicrobial activity, and may require an increase in dosage.

Volume of Distribution (V_d). Represents the apparent volume into which the drug is distributed, and is calculated as the amount of drug in the body divided by the serum concentration (in liters/kilogram). V_d is related to total body water distribution (V_d H_2O = 0.7 L/kg). Hydrophilic (water soluble) drugs are restricted to extracellular fluid and have a $V_d \leq 0.7$ L/kg. In contrast, hydrophobic (highly lipid soluble) drugs penetrate most fluids/tissues of the body and have a large V_d. Drugs that are concentrated in certain tissues (e.g., liver) can have a V_d greatly exceeding total body water. V_d is affected by organ profusion, membrane diffusion/permeability, lipid solubility, protein binding, and state of equilibrium between body compartments. For hydrophilic drugs, increases in V_d may occur with burns, heart failure, dialysis, sepsis, cirrhosis, or mechanical ventilation; decreases in V_d may occur with trauma, hemorrhage, pancreatitis (early), or GI fluid losses. Increases in V_d may require an increase in total daily drug dose for antimicrobial effectiveness; decreases in V_d may require a decrease in drug dose. In addition to drug distribution, V_d reflects binding avidity to cholesterol membranes and concentration within organ tissues (e.g., liver).

Mode of Elimination. Refers to the primary route of inactivation/excretion of the antibiotic, which impacts dosing adjustments in renal/hepatic failure.

Dosage Adjustments. Each grid provides dosing adjustments based on renal and hepatic function. Antimicrobial dosing for hemodialysis (HD)/peritoneal dialysis (PD) patients is the same as indicated for patients with a CrCl < 10 mL/min. Some antimicrobial agents require a supplemental dose immediately after hemodialysis (post–HD)/peritoneal dialysis (post–PD); following the supplemental dose, antimicrobial dosing should once again resume as indicated for a CrCl < 10 mL/min. "No change" indicates no change from the usual dose. "Avoid" indicates the drug should be avoided in the setting described. "None" indicates no supplemental dose is required. "No information" indicates there are insufficient data from which to make a dosing recommendation. Dosing recommendations are based on data, experience, or pharmacokinetic parameters. CVVH dosing recommendations represent general guidelines, since antibiotic removal is dependent on area/type of filter, ultrafiltration rates, and sieving coefficients; replacement dosing should be individualized and guided by serum levels, if possible. Creatinine clearance (CrCl) is used to gauge the degree of renal insufficiency, and can be estimated by the following calculation: CrCl (mL/min) = [(140 – age) x weight (kg)] / [72 x serum creatinine (mg/dL)]. The calculated value is multiplied by 0.85 for females. It is important to recognize that due to age-dependent decline in renal function, elderly patients with "normal" serum creatinines may have low CrCls requiring dosage adjustments. (For example, a 70-year-old, 50-kg female with a serum creatinine of 1.2 mg/dL has an estimated CrCl of 34 mL/min.) "Antiretroviral Dosage Adjustment" grids indicate recommended dosage adjustments when protease inhibitors (PIs) and non-nucleoside reverse transcriptase inhibitor (NNRTIs) are combined or used in conjunction with rifampin or rifabutin. These grids were compiled, in part, from "Guidelines for the Use of Antiretroviral Agents in HIV-Infected Adults and Adolescents," Panel on Clinical Practices for Treatment of HIV Infection, Department of Health and Human Services, www.aidsinfo.nih.gov/guidelines/. January 29, 2008.

Drug Interactions. Refers to common/important drug interactions, as compiled from various sources. If a specific drug interaction is well-documented, then other drugs from the same drug class (e.g., atorvastatin) may also be listed, based on theoretical considerations. Drug interactions may occur as a consequence of altered absorption (e.g., metal ion chelation of tetracycline), altered distribution (e.g., sulfonamide displacement of barbiturates from serum albumin), altered metabolism (e.g., rifampin–induced hepatic P-450 metabolism of theophylline/warfarin; chloramphenicol inhibition of phenytoin metabolism), or altered excretion (e.g., probenecid competition with penicillin for active transport in the kidney).

Adverse Side Effects. Common/important side effects are indicated.

Allergic Potential. Described as low or high. Refers to the likelihood of a hypersensitivity reaction to a particular antimicrobial.

Table 9.1. USFDA Use-in-Pregnancy Letter Code

Category	Interpretation
A	**Controlled studies show no risk.** Adequate, well-controlled studies in pregnant women have not shown a risk to the fetus in any trimester of pregnancy
B	**No evidence of risk in humans.** Adequate, well-controlled studies in pregnant women have not shown increased risk of fetal abnormalities despite adverse findings in animals, or, in the absence of adequate human studies, animal studies show no fetal risk. The chance of fetal harm is remote, but remains a possibility
C	**Risk cannot be ruled out.** Adequate, well-controlled human studies are lacking, and animal studies have shown a risk to the fetus or are lacking. There is a chance of fetal harm if the drug is administered during pregnancy, but potential benefit from use of the drug may outweigh potential risk
D	**Positive evidence of risk.** Studies in humans or investigational or post-marketing data have demonstrated fetal risk. Nevertheless, potential benefit from use of the drug may outweigh potential risk. For example, the drug may be acceptable if needed in a life-threatening situation or serious disease for which safer drugs cannot be used or are ineffective
X	**Contraindicated in pregnancy.** Studies in animals or humans or investigational or post-marketing reports have demonstrated positive evidence of fetal abnormalities or risk which clearly outweigh any possible benefit to the patient

Safety in Pregnancy. Designated by the U.S. Food and Drug Administration's (USFDA) use-in-pregnancy letter code (Table 9.1).

Antiretroviral Pregnancy Registry. To monitor maternal-fetal outcomes of pregnant women exposed to antiretroviral drugs, an Antiretroviral Pregnancy Registry has been established. Clinicians who are treating HIV-infected pregnant women are strongly encouraged to report cases of prenatal exposure to antiretroviral drugs (either administered alone or in combinations). The registry collects observational, non-experimental data regarding antiretroviral exposure during pregnancy for the purpose of assessing potential teratogenicity. Telephone: 910-251-9087 or 1-800-258-4263. Website: http://www.apregistry.com/who.htm

Comments. Includes various useful information for each antimicrobial agent.

Biliary Tract Penetration. Indicated as a percentage relative to peak serum concentrations. Percentages > 100% reflect concentration within the biliary system. This information is useful for the treatment of biliary tract infections.

Selected References. These references are classic, important, or recent. When available, the website containing the manufacturer's prescribing information/package insert is provided.

Abacavir (Ziagen) ABC

Drug Class: Antiretroviral NRTI (nucleoside reverse transcriptase inhibitor)
Usual Dose: 300 mg (PO) q12h
Pharmacokinetic Parameters:
Peak serum level: 3 mcg/mL
Bioavailability: 83%
Excreted unchanged (urine): 1.2%
Serum half-life (normal/ESRD): 1.5 /8 hrs
Plasma protein binding: 50%
Volume of distribution (V_d): 0.86 L/kg
Primary Mode of Elimination: Hepatic
Dosage Adjustments*

CrCl 50–80 mL/min	No change
CrCl 10–50 mL/min	No change
CrCl < 10 mL/min	No change
Post–HD dose	None
Post–PD dose	None
CVVH dose	No change
Mild hepatic insufficiency	200 mg (PO) q24h
Moderate or severe hepatic insufficiency	Avoid

Drug Interactions: Methadone (↑ methadone clearance with abacavir 600 mg bid); ethanol (↑ abacavir serum levels/half-life and may ↑ toxicity)
Adverse Effects: ***Abacavir may cause severe hypersensitivity reactions (see comments), usually during the first 4-6 weeks of therapy, which may be fatal;*** report cases of hypersensitivity syndrome to Abacavir Hypersensitivity Registry at 1-800-270-0425. Drug fever/rash, abdominal pain/diarrhea, nausea, vomiting, anorexia, insomnia, weakness, headache, ↑ SGOT/SGPT, hyperglycemia, hypertriglyceridemia, lactic acidosis with hepatic steatosis (rare, but potentially life-threatening toxicity with use of NRTI's)
Allergic Potential: High (~ 5%)
Safety in Pregnancy: C
Comments: May be taken with or without foods. Discontinue abacavir and ***do not restart in patients with signs/symptoms of hypersensitivity reaction***, which may include fever, rash, fatigue, nausea, vomiting, diarrhea, abdominal pain, anorexia, respiratory symptoms. Ethanol increases abacavir levels by 41%
Cerebrospinal Fluid Penetration: 27-33%

REFERENCES:

Carr A, Workman C, Smith DE, et al. Abacavir substitution for nucleoside analogs in patients with HIV lipoatrophy. A randomized trial. JAMA 288:207-15, 2002.
Cutrell A, Brothers C, Yeo J, et al. Abacavir and the potential risk of myocardial infarction. Lancet 2008 April1 1, e-pub.
Katalama C, Clotet B, Plettenberg A, et al. The role of abacavir (AVC, 1592) in antiretroviral therapy-experiences patients: results from randomized, double-blind, trial. CNA3002 European Study Team. AIDS 14:781-9, 2000.
Keating MR. Antiviral agents. Mayo Clin Proc 67:160-78, 1992.
Mallal S, Phillips E, Carosi G, et al. HLA-B*5701 screening for hypersensitivity to abacavir. N Engl J Med 358:568-79, 2008.
McDowell JA, Lou Y, Symonds WS, et al. Multiple-dose pharmacokinetics and pharmacodynamics of abacavir alone and in combination with zidovudine in human immunodeficiency virus-infected adults. Antimicrob Agents Chemother 44:2061-7, 2000.
Panel on Clinical Practices for Treatment of HIV Infection. Guidelines for the Use of Antiretroviral Agents in HIV-Infected Adults and Adolescents. Department of Health and Human Services. www.aidsinfo.nih.gov/guidelines/. Jan 29, 2008.
Staszewski S, Keiser P, Mantaner J, et al. Abacavir-lamivudine-zidovudine vs. indinavir-lamivudine-zidovudine in antiretroviral-naive HIV-infected adults: a randomized equivalence trial. JAMA 285:1155-63, 2001.
Website: www.TreatHIV.com

Abacavir + Lamivudine (Epzicom)

Drug Class: Antiretroviral NRTI combination
Usual Dose: Epzicom tablet = abacavir 600 mg + lamivudine 300 mg. Usual dose: 1 tablet q24h
Pharmacokinetic Parameters:
Peak serum level: 3/1.5 mcg/L

"Usual dose" assumes normal renal/hepatic function. * For renal insufficiency, give usual dose x 1 followed by maintenance dose per CrCl. For dialysis patients, dose the same as for CrCl < 10 mL/min and give supplemental (post-HD/PD dose) immediately after dialysis. CrCl = creatinine clearance; CVVH = continuous veno-venous hemofiltration; HD/PD = hemodialysis/peritoneal dialysis. See pp. 147-150 for explanations, p. 3 for abbreviations

Bioavailability: 83/86%
Excreted unchanged (urine): 1.2/71%
Serum half-life (normal/ESRD): (1.5/8)/(5-7/20) hrs
Plasma protein binding: 50/36%
Volume of distribution (V_d): 0.86/1.3 L/kg
Primary Mode of Elimination: Hepatic/Renal
Dosage Adjustments

CrCl < 50 mL/min	Not recommended
Post–HD dose	Not recommended
Post–PD dose	Not recommended
CVVH dose	Not recommended
Mild hepatic insufficiency	Contraindicated
Moderate or severe hepatic insufficiency	Contraindicated

Drug Interactions: Methadone (↑ methadone clearance with abacavir 600 mg bid); ethanol (↑ abacavir serum levels/half-life; may ↑ toxicity); didanosine, zalcitabine (↑ risk of pancreatitis); TMP-SMX (↑ lamivudine levels); zidovudine (↑ zidovudine levels)
Adverse Effects: Abacavir may cause severe hypersensitivity reaction that may be fatal (see comments), usually during the first 4-6 weeks of therapy; report cases of hypersensitivity reactions to Abacavir Hypersensitivity Registry at 1-800-270-0425. Drug fever, rash, abdominal pain, diarrhea, nausea, vomiting, anorexia, anemia, leukopenia, photophobia, depression, insomnia, weakness, headache, cough, nasal complaints, dizziness, peripheral neuropathy, myalgias, ↑ AST/ALT, hyperglycemia, hypertriglyceridemia, pancreatitis, lactic acidosis with hepatic steatosis (rare, but potentially life-threatening toxicity with the NRTI's)
Allergic Potential: High (~5%)/Low
Safety in Pregnancy: C
Comments: May be taken with or without food. **Discontinue and do not restart in patients with signs/symptoms of hypersensitivity reactions**, which may include fever, rash, fatigue, nausea, vomiting, diarrhea, abdominal pain, anorexia, respiratory symptoms. Potential cross-resistance with didanosine. Lamivudine prevents development of ZDV resistance and restores ZDV susceptibility. For patients co-infected with HIV and HBV, monitor hepatic function closely during therapy and for several months afterward
Cerebrospinal Fluid Penetration: 27-33/15%

REFERENCES:

No authors listed. Two once-daily fixed-dose NRTI combination for HIV. Med Lett Drugs Ther. 47:19-20, 2005.
Panel on Clinical Practices for Treatment of HIV Infection. Guidelines for the Use of Antiretroviral Agents in HIV-Infected Adults and Adolescents. Department of Health and Human Services. www.aidsinfo.nih.gov/guidelines/. Jan 29, 2008.
Sosa N, Hill-Zabala C, Dejesus E, et al. Abacavir and lamivudine fixed-dose combination tablet once daily compared with abacavir and lamivudine twice daily in HIV-infected patients over 48 weeks. J Acquir Immune Defic Syndr. 40:422-7, 2005.
Website: www.epzicom.com

Abacavir + Lamivudine + Zidovudine (Trizivir)

Drug Class: Antiretroviral NRTI combination
Usual Dose: Trizivir tablet = abacavir 300 mg + lamivudine 150 mg + zidovudine 300 mg. Usual dose = 1 tablet (PO) q12h
Pharmacokinetic Parameters:
Peak serum level: 3/1.5/1.2 mcg/mL
Bioavailability: 86/86/64%
Excreted unchanged (urine): 1.2/90/16%
Serum half-life (normal/ESRD): [1.5/6/1.1]/ 8/20/2.2] hrs
Plasma protein binding: 30/36/20%
Volume of distribution (V_d): 0.86/1.3/1.6 L/kg
Primary Mode of Elimination: Hepatic/renal
Dosage Adjustments*

CrCl < 50 mL/min	Avoid
Post–HD or post–PD	Avoid
CVVH dose	Avoid
Moderate or severe hepatic insufficiency	Not recommended

"Usual dose" assumes normal renal/hepatic function. * For renal insufficiency, give usual dose x 1 followed by maintenance dose per CrCl. For dialysis patients, dose the same as for CrCl < 10 mL/min and give supplemental (post-HD/PD dose) immediately after dialysis. CrCl = creatinine clearance; CVVH = continuous veno-venous hemofiltration; HD/PD = hemodialysis/peritoneal dialysis. See pp. 147-150 for explanations, p. 3 for abbreviations

Drug Interactions: Amprenavir, atovaquone (↑ zidovudine levels); clarithromycin (↓ zidovudine levels); cidofovir (↑ zidovudine levels, flu-like symptoms); doxorubicin (neutropenia); stavudine (antagonistic to zidovudine; avoid combination); TMP-SMX (↑ lamivudine and zidovudine levels); zalcitabine (↓ lamivudine levels)
Adverse Effects: ***Abacavir may cause severe/fatal rash/hypersensitivity reaction;*** do not restart after reaction. Must not be used in patients with prior abacavir reactions. Most common (>5%): nausea, vomiting, diarrhea, anorexia, insomnia, fever/chills, headache, malaise/fatigue. Others (less common): peripheral neuropathy, myopathy, steatosis, pancreatitis. Lab abnormalities: mild hyperglycemia, anemia, LFT elevations, hypertriglyceridemia, leukopenia
Allergic Potential: High (~5%)
Safety in Pregnancy: C
Comments: Avoid in patients with CrCl < 50 mL/min. May be taken with or without food. HBV hepatitis may relapse if lamivudine is discontinued

REFERENCES:
Havlir DV, Lange JM. New antiretrovirals and new combinations. AIDS 12(Suppl A):S165-74, 1998.
McDowell JA, Lou Y, Symonds WS, et al. Multiple-dose pharmacokinetics and pharmacodynamics of abacavir alone and in combination with zidovudine in human immunodeficiency virus-infected adults. Antimicrob Agents Chemother 44:2061-7, 2000.
Panel on Clinical Practices for Treatment of HIV Infection. Guidelines for the Use of Antiretroviral Agents in HIV-Infected Adults and Adolescents. Department of Health and Human Services. www.aidsinfo.nih.gov/guidelines/. Jan 29, 2008.
Three new drugs for HIV infection. Med Lett Drugs Ther 40:114-6, 1998.
Weverling GJ, Lange JM, Jurriaans S, et al. Alternative multidrug regimen provides improved suppression of HIV-1 replication over triple therapy. AIDS 12:117-22, 1998.
Website: www.TreatHIV.com

Adefovir dipivoxil (Hepsera)

Drug Class: Antihepatitis B agent
Usual Dose: 10 mg (PO) q24h

Pharmacokinetic Parameters:
Peak serum level: 18 ng/mL
Bioavailability: 59%
Excreted unchanged (urine): 45%
Serum half-life (normal/ESRD): 7.5/9 hrs
Plasma protein binding: 4%
Volume of distribution (V_d): 0.4 L/kg
Primary Mode of Elimination: Renal
Dosage Adjustments*

CrCl ≥ 50 mL/min	10 mg (PO) q24h
CrCl 20-50 mL/min	10 mg (PO) q48h
CrCl 10–20 mL/min	10 mg (PO) q72h
Hemodialysis	10 mg (PO) q7d
Post–HD or PD dose	No information
CVVH dose	No information
Moderate or severe hepatic insufficiency	No change

Drug Interactions: No significant interaction with lamivudine, TMP-SMX, acetaminophen, ibuprofen
Adverse Effects: Asthenia, headache, abdominal pain, nausea, flatulence, diarrhea, dyspepsia
Allergic Potential: Low
Safety in Pregnancy: C
Comments: May be taken with or without food. Does not inhibit CP450 isoenzymes. Do not discontinue abruptly to avoid exacerbation of HBV hepatitis
Cerebrospinal Fluid Penetration: No data

REFERENCES:
Buti M, Esteban R. Adefovir dipivoxil. Drugs of Today 39:127-35, 2003.
Cundy KC, Burditch-Crovo P, Walker RE, et al. Clinical pharmacokinetics of adefovir in human HIV-1 infected patients. Antimicrob Agents Chemother 35:2401-2405, 1995.
Davis GL. Update on the management of chronic hepatitis B. Rev Gastroenterol Disord 2:106-15, 2002.
Hadziyannis SJ, Tassopoulos NC, Heathcote E, et al. Adefovir dipivoxil for the treatment of hepatitis B e antigen-negative chronic hepatitis B. N Engl J Med 348:800-7, 2003.
Perillo R, Schiff E, Yoshida E, et al. Adefovir for the

"Usual dose" assumes normal renal/hepatic function. * For renal insufficiency, give usual dose x 1 followed by maintenance dose per CrCl. For dialysis patients, dose the same as for CrCl < 10 mL/min and give supplemental (post-HD/PD dose) immediately after dialysis. CrCl = creatinine clearance; CVVH = continuous veno-venous hemofiltration; HD/PD = hemodialysis/peritoneal dialysis. See pp. 147-150 for explanations, p. 3 for abbreviations

treatment of lamivudine-resistant hepatitis B mutants. Hepatology 32:129-34, 2000.
Peters MG, Hann Hw H, Martin P, et al. Adefovir dipivoxil alone or in combination with lamivudine in patients with lamivudine-resistant chronic hepatitis B. Gastroenterology 126:90-101, 2004.
Website: www.hepsera.com

Atazanavir (Reyataz) ATV

Drug Class: Antiretroviral protease inhibitor
Usual Dose: 400 mg (PO) q24h; 300 mg (PO) q24h when given with ritonavir 100 mg (PO) q24h
Pharmacokinetic Parameters:
Peak serum level: 3152 ng/mL
Bioavailability: No data
Excreted unchanged (urine) (urine/feces): 7%/20%
Serum half-life (normal/ESRD): 7 hrs/no data
Plasma protein binding: 86%
Volume of distribution (V_d): No data
Primary Mode of Elimination: Hepatic
Dosage Adjustments*

CrCl < 50 mL/min	No data
Post–HD or PD dose	No data
CVVH dose	No data
Moderate hepatic insufficiency	300 mg (PO) q24h
Severe hepatic insufficiency	Avoid

Antiretroviral Dosage Adjustments:

Delavirdine	No information
Didanosine	Give atazanavir 2 hrs before or 1 hr after didanosine buffered formulations
Efavirenz	Atazanavir 300 mg + ritonavir 100 + efavirenz 600 mg as single daily dose with food
Indinavir	Avoid combination
Lopinavir/ritonavir	No information
Nelfinavir	No information
Nevirapine	No information
Ritonavir	Atazanavir 300 mg/d + ritonavir 100 mg/d as single daily dose with food
Saquinavir	↑ saquinavir (soft-gel) levels; no information
Rifampin	Avoid combination
Rifabutin	150 mg q48h or 3x/week

Drug Interactions: Antacids or buffered medications (↓ atazanavir levels; give atazanavir 2 hours before or 1 hour after); H_2-receptor blockers (↓ atazanavir levels. In treatment-naive patients taking an H_2-receptor antagonist, give either atazanavir 400 mg once daily with food at least 2 hours before and at least 10 hours after the H_2-receptor antagonist, or give atazanavir 300 mg once daily with ritonavir 100 mg once daily with food, without the need for separation from the H_2-receptor antagonist. In treatment-experienced patients, give atazanavir 300 mg once daily with ritonavir 100 mg once daily with food at least 2 hours before and at least 10 hours after the H_2-receptor antagonist); antiarrhythmics (↑ amiodarone, systemic lidocaine, quinidine levels; prolongs PR interval; monitor antiarrhythmic levels); antidepressants (↑ tricyclic antidepressant levels; monitor levels); calcium channel blockers (↑ calcium channel blocker levels, ↑ PR interval; ↓ diltiazem dose by 50%; use with caution; consider ECG monitoring); clarithromycin (↑ clarithromycin and atazanavir levels; consider 50% dose reduction; consider alternate agent for infections not caused by MAI); cyclosporine, sirolimus, tacrolimus (↑ immunosuppressant levels; monitor levels); ethinyl estradiol, norethindrone (↑ oral contraceptive levels; use lowest effective oral contraceptive dose); lovastatin, simvastatin (↑ risk of myopathy,

"Usual dose" assumes normal renal/hepatic function. * For renal insufficiency, give usual dose x 1 followed by maintenance dose per CrCl. For dialysis patients, dose the same as for CrCl < 10 mL/min and give supplemental (post-HD/PD dose) immediately after dialysis. CrCl = creatinine clearance; CVVH = continuous veno-venous hemofiltration; HD/PD = hemodialysis/peritoneal dialysis. See pp. 147-150 for explanations, p. 3 for abbreviations

rhabdomyolysis; avoid combination); sildenafil (↑ sildenafil levels; do not give more than 25 mg q48h); tadalafil (max. 10 mg/72 hours); vardenafil (max. 2.5 mg/72 hours); St. John's wort (avoid combination); warfarin (↑ warfarin levels; monitor INR); tenofovir (tenofovir reduces systemic exposure to atazanavir. Whenever the two are co-administered, the recommended dose of atazanavir is 300 mg once daily with ritonavir 100 mg once daily). *Drugs that should not be co-administered with atazanavir* include beta-blockers, cisapride, pimozide, rifampin, irinotecan, midazolam, triazolam, lovastatin, simvastatin, bepridil, some ergot derivatives, indinavir, proton pump inhibitors, St. John's wort

Adverse Effects: Reversible, asymptomatic ↑ in indirect (unconjugated) bilirubin may occur. Asymptomatic, dose-dependent ↑ PR interval (~ 24 msec). Use with caution with drugs that ↑ PR interval (e.g., beta blockers, verapamil, digoxin). May ↑ risk of hyperglycemia/diabetes. May ↑ risk of bleeding in hemophilia (types A + B)

Allergic Potential: Low

Safety in Pregnancy: B

Comments: Monitor LFTs in patients with HBV, HCV. Take 400 mg (two 200-mg capsules) once daily with food

REFERENCES:

Colonno RJ, Thiry A, Limoli K, Parkin N. Activities of atazanavir (BMS-232632) against a large panel of Human Immunodeficiency Virus Type 1 clinical isolates resistant to one or more approved protease inhibitors. Antimicrob Agents Chemother 47:1324-33, 2003.

Haas DW, Zala C, Schrader S, et al. Therapy with atazanavir plus saquinavir in patients failing highly active antiretroviral therapy: a randomized comparative pilot trial. AIDS 17:1339-1349,2003.

Havlir DV, O'Marro SD. Atazanavir: new option for treatment of HIV infection. Clin Infect Dis 38:1599-604, 2004.

Jemsek JG, Arathoon E, Arlotti M, et al. Body fat and other metabolic effects of atazanavir and efavirenz, each administered in combination with zidovudine plus lamivudine, in antiretroviral-naive HIV-infected patients. Clin Infect Dis 42:273-80, 2006.

Panel on Clinical Practices for Treatment of HIV Infection. Guidelines for the Use of Antiretroviral Agents in HIV-Infected Adults and Adolescents. Department of Health and Human Services. www.aidsinfo.nih.gov/guidelines/. Jan 29, 2008.

Piliero PJ. Atazanavir: a novel HIV-1 protease inhibitor. Expert Opin Investig Drugs 11:1295-301, 2002.

Sanne I, Piliero P, Squires K, et al. Results of a phase 2 clinical trial at 48 weeks (AI424-007): a dose-ranging, safety, and efficacy comparative trial of atazanavir at three doses in combination with didanosine and stavudine in antiretroviral-naive subjects. J Acquir Immune Defic Syndr 32:18-29, 2003.

Wang F, Ross J. Atazanavir: a novel azapeptide inhibitor of HIV-1 protease. Formulary 38:691-702, 2003.

Website: www.reyataz.com

Darunavir (Prezista) DRV

Drug Class: Antiretroviral protease inhibitor

Usual Dose: 600 mg (two 300-mg tablets) of darunavir (PO) q12h plus 100 mg of ritonavir (PO) q12h

Pharmacokinetic Parameters:

Peak serum level: 3578 ng/mL

Bioavailability: 37% (alone) 82% (with ritonavir)

Excreted unchanged: 41.2% (feces), 7.7% (urine)

Serum half-life (normal/ESRD): 15/15 hrs

Plasma protein binding: 95%

Volume of distribution (V_d): not studied

Primary Mode of Elimination: Fecal/renal

Dosage Adjustments*

CrCl 50–80 mL/min	No change
CrCl 10–50 mL/min	No change
CrCl < 10 mL/min	No change
Post–HD dose	No change
Post–PD dose	No change
CVVH dose	No change
Mild hepatic insufficiency	Not studied
Moderate or severe hepatic insufficiency	Not studied

Antiretroviral Dosage Adjustments:

Efavirenz	No information
Nevirapine	No change

"Usual dose" assumes normal renal/hepatic function. * For renal insufficiency, give usual dose x 1 followed by maintenance dose per CrCl. For dialysis patients, dose the same as for CrCl < 10 mL/min and give supplemental (post-HD/PD dose) immediately after dialysis. CrCl = creatinine clearance; CVVH = continuous veno-venous hemofiltration; HD/PD = hemodialysis/peritoneal dialysis. See pp. 147-150 for explanations, p. 3 for abbreviations

Didanosine	1 hour before or 1 hour after darunavir
Tenofovir	No change
Fosamprenavir	No change
Indinavir	No information
Lopinavir/ritonavir	Avoid
Saquinavir	Avoid
Rifabutin	150 mg qod

Drug Interactions: Indinavir, ketaconazole, nevirapine, tenofovir (↑ darunavir levels); lopinavir/ritonavir, saquinavir, efavirenz (↓ darunavir levels); concomitant administration of darunavir/ritonavir with agents highly-dependent on CYP3A for clearance, astemizole, cisapride, dihydroergotamine, ergonovine, ergotamine, methylergonovine, midazolam, pimozide, terfenadine, midazolam, triazolam (may ↓ darunavir levels and ↓ effectiveness); sildenafil, vardenafil, tadalafil (↑ PDE-5 inhibitors; sildenafil do not exceed 25 mg in 48 hrs, vardenafil do not exceed 2.5 mg in 72 hrs, or tadalafil do not exceed 10 mg in 72 hrs)
Adverse Effects: Diarrhea, nausea, headache, nasopharyngitis
Allergic Potential: High (see comments)
Safety in Pregnancy: B
Comments: Always take with food (increases AUC, Cmax by approximately 30%). Must be given with ritonavir to boost bioavailability. Darunavir contains a sulfonamide moiety (as do fosamprenavir and tipranavir); use with caution in patients with sulfonamide allergies. A mild-to-moderate rash occurred in 7% of patients receiving the drug in clinical trial, it did not usually require drug cessation, but severe rashes (including Stevens-Johnson syndrome) have been reported
Cerebrospinal Fluid Penetration: No data

REFERENCES:

Clotet B, Bellos N, Moloina JM, et al. Efficacy and safety of darunavir-ritonavir at week 48 in treatment-experienced patients with HIV-1 infection in POWER 1 and 2: a pooled subgroup analysis of data from two randomised trials. Lancet 369:1169-78, 2007.

De Meyer S, Azijn H, Surleraux D, et al. TMC114, a novel human immunodeficiency virus type 1 protease inhibitor active against protease inhibitor-resistant viruses, including a broad range of clinical isolates. Antimicrobial Agents & Chemotherapy 2005;49:2314-2321.

Dominique L. N. G, Surleraux T, Abdellah Tahri T, et al. Discovery and selection of TMC114, a next generation HIV-I protease inhibitor. J. Med. Chem. 2005;48:1813-1822.

Grinsztejn, B. TMC114/r is well tolerated in 3-class-experienced patients: week 24 of POWER 1 (TMC114-C213). Tibotec Pharmaceuticals. Rio de Janerio, Brazil. Available from URL: http://www.tibotec.com/content/congresses/www.tibotec.com/TMC114_SafetyPoster_Dr_Grinsztein_IAS_FINAL.pdf.

Katlama C. TMC114/r outperforms investigator-selected PI(s) in 3-class-experienced patients: week 24 primary efficacy analysis of POWER 1 (TMC114-C213). Tibotec Pharmaceuticals. Rio de Janerio, Brazil. Available from URL: http://www.tibotec.com/content/congresses/www.tibotec.com/TMC114_EfficacyPoster_ProfKatlama_Finalias2005.pdf

Madruga JV, Berger D, McMurchie M, et al. Efficacy and safety of darunavir-ritonavir compared with that of lopinavir-ritonavir at 48 weeks in treatment-experienced, HIV-infected patients in TITAN: a randomised controlled phase III trial. Lancet 370:3-5, 2007.

Product Information: PREZISTA(TM) oral tablets, darunavir oral tablets. Tibotec Therapeutics, Inc, Raritan, NJ, 2006.

Sorbera LA, Castaner J, Bayes M. Darunavir: Anti-HIV agent HIV protease inhibitor. Drugs of the Future. 2005;30:441-449.

Website: www.prezista.com

Delavirdine (Rescriptor)

Drug Class: Antiretroviral NNRTI (non-nucleoside reverse transcriptase inhibitor)
Usual Dose: 400 mg (PO) q8h
Pharmacokinetic Parameters:
Peak serum level: 35 mcg/mL
Bioavailability: 85%
Excreted unchanged (urine): 5%
Serum half-life (normal/ESRD): 5.8 hrs/no data
Plasma protein binding: 98%
Volume of distribution (V_d): 0.5 L/kg
Primary Mode of Elimination: Hepatic

Dosage Adjustments*

CrCl 50–80 mL/min	No change
CrCl 10–50 mL/min	No change
CrCl < 10 mL/min	No change
Post–HD dose	None
Post–PD dose	None
CVVH dose	No change
Moderate hepatic insufficiency	No information
Severe hepatic insufficiency	No information

Antiretroviral Dosage Adjustments:

Efavirenz	No information
Indinavir	Indinavir 600 mg q8h
Lopinavir/ritonavir	No information
Nelfinavir	No information (monitor for neutropenia)
Nevirapine	No information
Ritonavir	Delavirdine: no change; ritonavir: No information
Saquinavir soft-gel	Saquinavir soft-gel 800 mg q8h (monitor transaminases)
Rifampin, rifabutin	Avoid combination
Statins	Not recommended

Drug Interactions: Antiretrovirals, rifabutin, rifampin (see dose adjustment grid, above); astemizole, terfenadine, benzodiazepines, cisapride, H_2 blockers, proton pump inhibitors, ergot alkaloids, quinidine, statins (avoid if possible); carbamazepine, phenobarbital, phenytoin (may ↓ delavirdine levels, monitor anticonvulsant levels); clarithromycin, dapsone, nifedipine, warfarin (↑ interacting drug levels); sildenafil (do not exceed 25 mg in 48 hrs); tadalafil (max. 10 mg/72 hrs); vardenafil (max. 2.5 mg/72 hrs)
Adverse Effects: Drug fever/rash, Stevens–Johnson syndrome (rare), headache, nausea/vomiting, diarrhea, ↑ SGOT/SGPT
Allergic Potential: High
Safety in Pregnancy: C
Comments: May be taken with or without food, but food decreases absorption by 20%. May disperse four 100-mg tablets in > 3 oz. water to produce slurry; 200-mg tablets should be taken as intact tablets and not used to make an oral solution. Separate dosing with ddI or antacids by 1 hour
Cerebrospinal Fluid Penetration: 0.4%

REFERENCES:

Been-Tiktak AM, Boucher CA, Brun-Vezinet F, et al. Efficacy and safety of combination therapy with delavirdine and zidovudine: A European/Australian phase II trial. Intern J Antimcrob Agents 11:13-21, 1999.

Conway B. Initial therapy with protease inhibitor-sparing regimens: Evaluation of nevirapine and delavirdine. Clin Infect Dis 2:130-4, 2000.

Demeter LM, Shafer RW, Meehan PM, et al. Delavirdine susceptibilities and associated reverse transcriptase mutations in human immunodeficiency virus type 1 isolates from patients in a phase I/II trial of delavirdine monotherapy (ACTG260). Antimicrob Agents Chemother 44:794-7, 2000.

Justesen US, Klitgaard NA, Brosen K, et al. Dose-dependent pharmacokinetics of delavirdine in combination with amprenavir in healthy volunteers. J Antimicrob Chemother 54:206-10, 2004.

Panel on Clinical Practices for Treatment of HIV Infection. Guidelines for the use of antiretroviral agents in HIV-infected adults and adolescents. Department of Health and Human Services. www.aidsinfo.nih.gov/guidelines/. Jan 29, 2008.

Website: rescriptor.com

Didanosine (Videx) ddI

Drug Class: Antiretroviral NRTI (nucleoside reverse transcriptase inhibitor)
Usual Dose: 400 mg q24h for weight > 60 kg; 250 mg q24h for < 60 kg
Pharmacokinetic Parameters:
Peak serum level: 29 mcg/mL

"Usual dose" assumes normal renal/hepatic function. * For renal insufficiency, give usual dose x 1 followed by maintenance dose per CrCl. For dialysis patients, dose the same as for CrCl < 10 mL/min and give supplemental (post-HD/PD dose) immediately after dialysis. CrCl = creatinine clearance; CVVH = continuous veno-venous hemofiltration; HD/PD = hemodialysis/peritoneal dialysis. See pp. 147-150 for explanations, p. 3 for abbreviations

Bioavailability: 42%
Excreted unchanged (urine): 60%
Serum half-life (normal/ESRD): 1.6/4.1 hrs
Plasma protein binding: ≤ 5%
Volume of distribution (V_d): 1.1 L/kg
Primary Mode of Elimination: Renal
Dosage Adjustments*: > 60 kg/[< 60 kg]:

CrCl 30–59 mL/min	200 mg (PO) q24h [125 mg (PO) q24h]
CrCl 10–29 mL/min	125 mg (PO) q24h [125 mg (PO) q24h]
CrCl < 10 mL/min	125 mg (PO) q24h [not recommended]
Post–HD dose	No information
Post–PD dose	100 mg (PO)
CVVH dose	150 mg (PO) q24h
Moderate hepatic insufficiency	No change
Severe hepatic insufficiency	No change

Drug Interactions: Alcohol, lamivudine, pentamidine, valproic acid (↑ risk of pancreatitis); dapsone, fluoroquinolones, ketoconazole, itraconazole, tetracyclines (↓ absorption of interacting drug; give 2 hours after didanosine); dapsone, INH, metronidazole, nitrofurantoin, stavudine, vincristine, zalcitabine, neurotoxic drugs or history of neuropathy (↑ risk of neuropathy); dapsone (↓ dapsone absorption, which increases risk of PCP); tenofovir (if possible, avoid concomitant tenofovir due to impaired CD4 response and increased risk of virologic failure). Avoid ribavirin in HIV patients
Adverse Effects: Headache, depression, nausea, vomiting, GI upset/abdominal pain, diarrhea, drug fever/rash, anemia, leukopenia, thrombocytopenia, hepatotoxicity/hepatic necrosis, pancreatitis (may be fatal; ↑ risk in patients on concomitant tenofovir), hypertriglyceridemia, hyperuricemia, lactic acidosis, lipoatrophy, wasting, dose-dependent (≥ 0.06 mg/kg/d) peripheral neuropathy, hyperglycemia, lactic acidosis with hepatic steatosis (rare, but potentially life-threatening toxicity with use of NRTI's; ***pregnant women taking didanosine + stavudine may be at increased risk***)
Allergic Potential: Low
Safety in Pregnancy: B; should be avoided in pregnancy as it may cause fatal pancreatitis
Comments: Available as buffered powder for oral solution and enteric-coated extended-release capsules (Videx EC 400 mg PO q24h). Take 30 minutes before or 2 hours after meal (food decreases serum concentrations by 49%). Avoid in patients with alcoholic cirrhosis/history of pancreatitis. Use with caution with ribavirin. Na^+ content = 11.5 mEq/g. Buffered tablets discontinued by US manufacturer in February 2006
Cerebrospinal Fluid Penetration: 20%

REFERENCES:

Barreiro P, Corbaton A, Nunez M, et al. Tolerance of didanosine as enteric-coated capsules versus buffered tablets. AIDS Patient Care STDS 18:329-31, 2004.
Hirsch MS, D'Aquila RT. Therapy for human immunodeficiency virus infection. N Engl J Med 328:1686-95, 1993.
HIV Trialists' Collaborative Group. Zidovudine, didanosine, and zalcitabine in the treatment of HIV infection: Meta-analyses of the randomised evidence. Lancet 353:2014-2025, 1999.
Montaner JS, Reiss P, Cooper D, et al. A randomized, double-blind trial comparing combinations of nevirapine, didanosine, and zidovudine for HIV-infected patients: The INCAS trial. Italy, the Netherlands, Canada and Australia Study. J Am Med Assoc 279:930-937, 1998.
Negredo E, Molto J, Munoz-Moreno JA, et al. Safety and efficacy of once-daily didanosine, tenofovir and nevirapine as a simplification antiretroviral approach. Antivir Ther 9:335-42, 2004.
Panel on Clinical Practices for Treatment of HIV Infection. Guidelines for the use of antiretroviral agents in HIV-infected adults and adolescents. Department of Health and Human Services. www.aidsinfo.nih.gov/guidelines/. Jan 29, 2008.
Perry CM, Balfour JA. Didanosine: An update on its antiviral activity, pharmacokinetic properties, and therapeutic efficacy in the management of HIV disease. Drugs 52:928-62, 1996.
Rathbun RC, Martin ES 3rd. Didanosine therapy in

"Usual dose" assumes normal renal/hepatic function. * For renal insufficiency, give usual dose x 1 followed by maintenance dose per CrCl. For dialysis patients, dose the same as for CrCl < 10 mL/min and give supplemental (post-HD/PD dose) immediately after dialysis. CrCl = creatinine clearance; CVVH = continuous veno-venous hemofiltration; HD/PD = hemodialysis/peritoneal dialysis. See pp. 147-150 for explanations, p. 3 for abbreviations

patients intolerant of or failing zidovudine therapy. Ann Pharmacother 26:1347-51, 1992.
Website: www.pdr.net

Efavirenz (Sustiva) EFV

Drug Class: Antiretroviral NNRTI (non-nucleoside reverse transcriptase inhibitor)
Usual Dose: 600 mg (PO) q24h
Pharmacokinetic Parameters:
Peak serum level: 12.9 mcg/mL
Bioavailability: Increased with food
Excreted unchanged (urine): 14-34%
Serum half-life (normal/ESRD): 40-55 hrs/no data
Plasma protein binding: 99%
Volume of distribution (V_d): No data
Primary Mode of Elimination: Hepatic
Dosage Adjustments*

CrCl < 60 mL/min	No change
Post–HD or PD dose	None
CVVH dose	No change
Moderate or severe hepatic insufficiency	No information

Antiretroviral Dosage Adjustments:

Delavirdine	No information
Indinavir	Indinavir 1000 mg q8h
Lopinavir/ ritonavir (l/r)	Consider l/r 533/133 mg q12h in PI-experienced patients
Nelfinavir	No changes
Nevirapine	No information
Ritonavir	Ritonavir 600 mg q12h (500 mg q12h for intolerance)
Saquinavir	Avoid use as sole PI
Rifampin	No changes
Rifabutin	Rifabutin 450-600 mg q24h or 600 mg 2-3x/week if not on protease inhibitor

Drug Interactions: Antiretrovirals, rifabutin, rifampin (see dose adjustment grid, above); astemizole, terfenadine, cisapride, ergotamine, midazolam, triazolam (avoid); carbamazepine, phenobarbital, phenytoin (monitor anticonvulsant levels; use with caution); caspofungin (↓ caspofungin levels, may ↓ caspofungin effect); methadone, clarithromycin (↓ interacting drug levels; titrate methadone dose to effect; consider using azithromycin instead of clarithromycin)
Adverse Effects: Drug fever/rash, CNS symptoms (nightmares, dizziness, neuropsychiatric symptoms, difficulty concentrating, somnolence), ↑ SGOT/SGPT, E. multiforme/Stevens–Johnson syndrome (rare), false positive cannabinoid test
Allergic Potential: High
Safety in Pregnancy: D
Comments: Rash/CNS symptoms usually resolve spontaneously over 2-4 weeks. Take at bedtime. Avoid taking after high fat meals (levels ↑ 50%). 600-mg dose available as single tablet
Cerebrospinal Fluid Penetration: 1%

REFERENCES:

Albrecht MA, Bosch RJ, Hammer SM, et al. Nelfinavir, efavirenz, or both after the failure of nucleoside treatment of HIV infection. N Engl J Med 345:398-407, 2001.
Gallant JE, DeJesus D, Arribas JR, et al. Tenofovir DF, emtricitabine, and efavirenz vs. zidovudine, lamivudine, and efavirenz for HIV. N Engl J Med 354:251-60, 2006.
Go JC, Cunha BA. Efavirenz. Antibiotics for Clinicians 5:1-8, 2001.
Haas DW, Fessel WJ, Delapenha RA, et al. Therapy with efavirenz plus indinavir in patients with extensive prior nucleoside reverse-transcriptase inhibitor experience: A randomized, double-blind, placebo-controlled trial. J Infect Dis 183:392-400, 2001.
la Porte CJ, de Graaff-Teulen MJ, Colbers EP, et al. Effect of efavirenz treatment on the pharmacokinetics of nelfinavir boosted by ritonavir in healthy volunteers. Br J Clin Pharmacol 58:632-40, 2004.
Marzolini C, Telenti A, Decosterd LA, et al. Efavirenz plasma levels can predict treatment failure and central nervous system side effects in HIV-1-infected patients. AIDS 15:71-5, 2001.
Negredo E, Cruz L, Paredes R, et al. Virological, immunological, and clinical impact of switching from protease inhibitors to nevirapine or to efavirenz in patients with human immunodeficiency virus infection

"Usual dose" assumes normal renal/hepatic function. * For renal insufficiency, give usual dose x 1 followed by maintenance dose per CrCl. For dialysis patients, dose the same as for CrCl < 10 mL/min and give supplemental (post-HD/PD dose) immediately after dialysis. CrCl = creatinine clearance; CVVH = continuous veno-venous hemofiltration; HD/PD = hemodialysis/peritoneal dialysis. See pp. 147-150 for explanations, p. 3 for abbreviations

and long-lasting viral suppression. Clin Infect Dis 34:504-510, 2002.
Panel on Clinical Practices for Treatment of HIV Infection. Guidelines for the use of antiretroviral agents in HIV-infected adults and adolescents. Department of Health and Human Services. www.aidsinfo.nih.gov/guidelines/. Jan 29, 2008.
Website: www.sustiva.com

Efavirenz + Emtricitabine + Tenofovir disoproxil fumarate (ATRIPLA)

Drug Class: Antiretroviral agent
Usual Dose: 1 tablet (efavirenz 600 mg/emtricitabine 200 mg/tenofovir 300 mg) (PO) q24h on an empty stomach
Pharmacokinetic Parameters:
Peak serum level: 4.0/1.8 mcg/mL/296 ng/mL
Bioavailability: NR/93%/25%
Excreted unchanged: < 1% unchanged and 14-30% as metabolites/86%/32%
Serum half-life (normal/ESRD): (40-55 hrs/~10 hrs on hemodialysis)/(10 hrs/extended)/(17 hrs/no data)
Plasma protein binding: 99/< 4/< 0.7%
Volume of distribution (V_d): NR/NR/1.2 L/kg
Primary Mode of Elimination: hepatic/renal/renal
Dosage Adjustments*

CrCl 50-80 mL/min	No change
CrCl 10-50 mL/min	Avoid
CrCl < 10 mL/min	Avoid
Post–HD dose	Avoid
Post–PD dose	Avoid
CVVH dose	Avoid
Mild hepatic insufficiency	No information
Moderate or severe hepatic insufficiency	No information

Antiretroviral Dosage Adjustments:

Fosamprenavir/ritonavir	An additional 100 mg/day (300 mg total) of ritonavir is recommended when ATRIPLA is administered with fosamprenavir/ritonavir q24h. No change in ritonavir dose when ATRIPLA is administered with fosamprenavir/ritonavir q12h
Atazanavir	Avoid
Indinavir	Indinavir 1000 mg q8h
Lopinavir/ritonavir	Increase lopinavir/ritonavir to 600/150 mg (3 tablets) q12h
Ritonavir	No information
Saquinavir	Avoid
Didanosine	Avoid
Rifabutin	Rifabutin 450-600 mg q24h or 600 mg 2-3x/week if not on protease inhibitor
Rifampin	No change

Drug Interactions: Antiretrovirals, rifabutin (see dose adjustment grid above); astemizole, cisapride, ergotamine, methylergonovine, midazolam, triazolam, St John's Wort (↓ efavirenz levels), voriconazole (↓ voriconazole levels; avoid); caspofungin (↓ caspofungin levels); carbamazepine, phenytoin, phenobarbital (monitor anticonvulsant levels; use with caution; potential for ↓ efavirenz levels); statins (may ↓ statin levels); methadone, (↓ methadone levels); clarithromycin (may ↓ clarithromycin effectiveness, consider using azithromycin)
Adverse Effects: Headache, diarrhea, nausea, vomiting, GI upset, lactic acidosis, osteopenia, rash, dizziness, fatigue, lactic acidosis with hepatic steatosis (rare but potentially life-threatening with NRTI's), relapsing type B viral hepatitis, depression, vivid dreams, renal impairment
Allergic Potential: High

"Usual dose" assumes normal renal/hepatic function. * For renal insufficiency, give usual dose x 1 followed by maintenance dose per CrCl. For dialysis patients, dose the same as for CrCl < 10 mL/min and give supplemental (post-HD/PD dose) immediately after dialysis. CrCl = creatinine clearance; CVVH = continuous veno-venous hemofiltration; HD/PD = hemodialysis/peritoneal dialysis. See pp. 147-150 for explanations, p. 3 for abbreviations

Safety in Pregnancy: D
Comments: Rash/CNS effects usually resolve in a few weeks. Take at bedtime on empty stomach. High fat meals can ↑ efavirenz by 50%. Use with caution in patients with history of seizures (↑ risk of convulsions). Potential for cross-resistance to lamivudine, zalcitabine, abacavir, and didanosine. Low affinity for DNA polymerase-gamma
Cerebrospinal Fluid Penetration: 1%/no data/no data

REFERENCES:

Gallant JE, DeJesus E, Arribas JR, et al: Tenofovir DF, emtricitabine, and efavirenz vs. zidovudine, lamivudine, and efavirenz for HIV. N Engl J Med 2006;354:251-260.

Izzedine H, Aymard G, Launay-Vacher V, et al. Pharmacokinetics of efavirenz in a patient on maintenance haemodialysis. AIDS 2000;14:618-619.

Panel on Clinical Practices for the Treatment of HIV Infection: Guidelines for the use of antiretroviral agents in HIV-1-infected adults and adolescents. Department of Health and Human Services. http://aidsinfo.nih.gov/ContentFiles/AdultandAdolescentGL.pdf. Jan 29, 2008.

ter Hofstede HJ, de Marie S, Foudraine NA. Clinical features and risk factors of lactic acidosis following long-term antiretroviral therapy: 4 fatal cases. Intl J STD AIDS 2000;11:611-616.

Website: www.atripla.com

Emtricitabine (Emtriva) FTC

Drug Class: Antiretroviral NRTI (nucleoside reverse transcriptase inhibitor)
Usual Dose: 200 mg (PO) q24h
Pharmacokinetic Parameters:
Peak serum level: 1.8 mcg/mL
Bioavailability: 93%
Excreted unchanged (urine): 86%
Serum half-life (normal/ESRD): 10 hrs/extended
Plasma protein binding: 4%
Primary Mode of Elimination: Renal
Dosage Adjustments*

CrCl ≥ 50 mL/min	200 mg (PO) q24h
CrCl 30-49 mL/min	200 mg (PO) q48h
CrCl 15-29 mL/min	200 mg (PO) q72h
CrCl < 15 mL/min	200 mg (PO) q96h
Post–HD dose	200 mg (PO) q96h
Post–PD dose	No information
CVVH dose	No information
Moderate or severe hepatic insufficiency	No change

Drug Interactions: No significant interactions with indinavir, stavudine, zidovudine, famciclovir, tenofovir
Adverse Effects: Headache, diarrhea, nausea, rash, lactic acidosis with hepatic steatosis (rare, but potentially life-threatening with NRTI's)
Allergic Potential: Low
Safety in Pregnancy: B
Comments: May be taken with or without food. Does not inhibit CYP450 enzymes. Mean intracellular half-live of 39 hours. Potential cross-resistance to lamivudine and zalcitabine. Low affinity for DNA polymerase-gamma.
Cerebrospinal Fluid Penetration: No data

REFERENCES:

Anderson PL. Pharmacologic perspectives for once-daily antiretroviral therapy. Ann Pharmacother 38:1924-34, 2004.

Benson CA, van der Horst C, Lamarca A, et al. A randomized study of emtricitabine and lamivudine in stable suppressed patients with HIV. AIDS 18:2269-2276, 2004.

Dando TM, Wagstaff AJ. Emtricitabine/tenofovir disoproxil fumarate. Drugs 64:2075-82, 2004.

Gallant JE, DeJesus D, Arribas JR, et al. Tenofovir DF, emtricitabine, and efavirenz vs. zidovudine, lamivudine, and efavirenz for HIV. N Engl J Med 354:251-60, 2006.

Lim SG, Ng TN, Kung N, et al. A double-blind placebo-controlled study of emtricitabine in chronic hepatitis B. Arch Intern Med 166:49-56, 2006.

Panel on Clinical Practices for Treatment of HIV Infection. Guidelines for the Use of Antiretroviral Agents in HIV-Infected Adults and Adolescents. Department of Health and Human Services. www.aidsinfo.nih.gov/guidelines/. Jan 29, 2008.

Saag MS. Emtricitabine, a new antiretroviral agent with activity against HIV and hepatitis B virus. Clin Infect Dis 42;128-31, 2006.

Website: www.emtriva.com

"Usual dose" assumes normal renal/hepatic function. * For renal insufficiency, give usual dose x 1 followed by maintenance dose per CrCl. For dialysis patients, dose the same as for CrCl < 10 mL/min and give supplemental (post-HD/PD dose) immediately after dialysis. CrCl = creatinine clearance; CVVH = continuous veno-venous hemofiltration; HD/PD = hemodialysis/peritoneal dialysis. See pp. 147-150 for explanations, p. 3 for abbreviations

Emtricitabine + Tenofovir disoproxil fumarate (Truvada)

Drug Class: Antiretroviral NRTI (nucleoside reverse transcriptase inhibitor) + nucleotide analogue
Usual Dose: One tablet (PO) q24h (each tablet contains 200 mg of emtricitabine + 300 mg of tenofovir)
Pharmacokinetic Parameters:
Peak serum level: 1.8/0.3 mcg/L
Bioavailability: 93%/27% if fasting (39% with high fat meal)
Excreted unchanged (urine): 86/32%
Serum half-life (normal/ESRD): (10 hrs/extended)/(17 hrs/no data)
Plasma protein binding: 4/0.7-7.2%
Volume of distribution (V_d): no data/1.3 L/kg
Primary Mode of Elimination: Renal/Renal
Dosage Adjustments*

CrCl ≥ 50 mL/min	No change
CrCl 30-49 mL/min	One capsule (PO) q48h
CrCl 15-29 mL/min	Avoid
CrCl < 15 mL/min	Avoid
Post–HD dose	Avoid
Post–PD dose	Avoid
CVVH dose	Avoid
Moderate or severe hepatic insufficiency	No change

Drug Interactions: No significant interactions with indinavir, stavudine, zidovudine, famciclovir, lamivudine, lopinavir/ritonavir, efavirenz, methadone, oral contraceptives. Tenofovir ↑ didanosine levels. Tenofovir reduces systemic exposure to atazanavir; whenever the two are co-administered, the recommended dose of atazanavir is 300 mg once daily with ritonavir 100 mg once daily
Adverse Effects: Headache, diarrhea, nausea, vomiting, GI upset, rash, lactic acidosis with hepatic steatosis (rare but potentially life-threatening with NRTI's)
Allergic Potential: Low
Safety in Pregnancy: B
Comments: May be taken with or without food. Does not inhibit CYP450 enzymes. Mean intracellular half-life with emtricitabine is 39 hours. Potential cross-resistance to lamivudine, zalcitabine, abacavir, didanosine. Low affinity for DNA polymerase-gamma. Avoid coadministration with didanosine
Cerebrospinal Fluid Penetration: No data

REFERENCES:

Dando TM, Wagstaff AJ. Emtricitabine/tenofovir disoproxil fumarate. Drugs 64:2075-82, 2004.
Gallant JE, DeJesus D, Arribas JR, et al. Tenofovir DF, emtricitabine, and efavirenz vs. zidovudine, lamivudine, and efavirenz for HIV. N Engl J Med 354:251-60, 2006.
Panel on Clinical Practices for Treatment of HIV Infection. Guidelines for the Use of Antiretroviral Agents in HIV-Infected Adults and Adolescents. Department of Health and Human Services. www.aidsinfo.nih.gov/guidelines/. Jan 29, 2008.
Website: www.truvada.com

Enfuvirtide (Fuzeon) ENF

Drug Class: Antiretroviral fusion inhibitor
Usual Dose: 90 mg (SC) q12h
Pharmacokinetic Parameters:
Peak serum level: 4.9 mcg/mL
Bioavailability: 84.3%
Serum half-life (normal/ESRD): 3.8 hrs/no data
Plasma protein binding: 92%
Volume of distribution (V_d): 5.5 L
Primary Mode of Elimination: Metabolized
Dosage Adjustments*

CrCl > 35 mL/min	No change
CrCl < 35 mL/min	No data
Post–HD dose	No data
Post–PD dose	No data
CVVH dose	No data

"Usual dose" assumes normal renal/hepatic function. * For renal insufficiency, give usual dose x 1 followed by maintenance dose per CrCl. For dialysis patients, dose the same as for CrCl < 10 mL/min and give supplemental (post-HD/PD dose) immediately after dialysis. CrCl = creatinine clearance; CVVH = continuous veno-venous hemofiltration; HD/PD = hemodialysis/peritoneal dialysis. See pp. 147-150 for explanations, p. 3 for abbreviations

Moderate or severe hepatic insufficiency	No data

Drug Interactions: No clinically significant interactions with other antiretrovirals. Does not inhibit CYP450 enzymes

Adverse Effects: Local injection site reactions are common. Diarrhea, nausea, fatigue may occur. Laboratory abnormalities include mild/transient eosinophilia. Pneumonia may occur, but cause is unclear and may not be due to drug therapy. Pancreatitis, myalgia, conjunctivitis (rare)

Allergic Potential: Hypersensitivity reactions may occur, including fever, chills, hypotension, rash, ↑ serum transaminases. Do not rechallenge following a hypersensitivity reaction

Safety in Pregnancy: B

Comments: Enfuvirtide interferes with entry of HIV-1 into cells by blocking fusion of HIV-1 and CD4 cellular membranes by binding to HR1 in the gp41 subunit of the HIV-1 envelope glycoprotein. Additive/synergistic with NRTI's, NNRTI's, and PI's, and no cross resistance to other antiretrovirals in cell culture. Compared to background regimen, enfuvirtide ↑ CD4 (71 vs. 35 cells/mm^3) and ↓ HIV-1 RNA (–1.52 $\log_{10}$ vs. –0.73 $\log_{10}$ copies/mL) at 24 weeks. Reconstitute in 1.1 mL of sterile water. SC injection should be given into upper arm, anterior thigh, or abdomen. Rotate injection sites; do not inject into moles, scars, bruises. After reconstitution, use immediately or refrigerate and use within 24 hours (no preservatives added)

REFERENCES:

Coleman CI, Musial, BL, Ross, J. Enfuvirtide: the first fusion inhibitor for the treatment of patients with HIV-1 infection. Formulary 38:204-222, 2003.

Kilby JM, Lalezari JP, Eron JJ, et al. The safety, plasma pharmacokinetics, and antiviral activity of subcutaneous enfuvirtide (T-20), a peptide inhibitor of gp41-mediated virus fusion, in HIV-infected adults. AIDS Res Hum Retroviruses 18:685-93, 2002.

Lalezari JP, Eron JJ, Carlson M, et al. A phase II clinical study of the long-term safety and antiviral activity of enfuvirtide-based antiretroviral therapy. AIDS 17:691-8, 2003.

Lalezari JP, Henry K, O'Hearn M, et al. TORO 1 Study Group. Enfuvirtide, an HIV-1 fusion inhibitor, for drug-resistant HIV infection in North and South America. N Engl J Med 348:2175-85, 2003.

Lazzarin A, Clotet B, Cooper D, et al. TORO 2 Study Group. Efficacy of enfuvirtide in patients infected with drug-resistant HIV-1 in Europe and Australia. N Engl J Med 348:2186-95, 2003.

Leao J, Frezzini C, Porter S. Enfuvirtide: a new class of antiretroviral therapy for HIV infection. Oral Dis 10:327-9, 2004.

Leen C, Wat C, Nieforth K. Pharmacokinetics of enfuvirtide in a patient with impaired renal function. Clin Infect Dis 4:339-55, 2004.

Panel on Clinical Practices for Treatment of HIV Infection. Guidelines for the Use of Antiretroviral Agents in HIV-Infected Adults and Adolescents. Department of Health and Human Services. www.aidsinfo.nih.gov/guidelines/. Jan 29, 2008.

Website: www.fuzeon.com

Etravirine (Intelence) ETR

Drug Class: Antiretroviral NNRTI (non-nucleoside reverse transcriptase inhibitor)

Usual Dose: 200 mg (PO) q12h following a meal

Pharmacokinetic Parameters:

Peak serum level: 296 ng/mL

Bioavailability: unknown (food increases systemic exposure)

Excreted unchanged: 81-86% (feces); 0% (urine)

Serum half-life (normal/ESRD): 41 hrs/not studied

Plasma protein binding: 99.9%

Volume of distribution (V_d): Not studied

Primary Mode of Elimination: Fecal 93.7%/renal 1.2%

Dosage Adjustments*

CrCl 50-80 mL/min	Not studied
CrCl 10-50 mL/min	Not studied
CrCl < 10 mL/min	Not studied
Post–HD dose	No change
Post–PD dose	No change
CVVH dose	Not studied

Moderate or severe hepatic insufficiency	No change
Co-infection with Hepatitis B or C virus	No change

Antiretroviral Dosage Adjustments:

Atazanavir/ritonavir	Avoid
Delavirdine	Avoid (↑ etravirine)
Efavirenz/nevirapine	Avoid (↓ etravirine)
Fosamprenavir/ritonavir	Use with caution (↑ amprenavir)
Lopinavir/ritonavir	Use with caution (↑ etravirine)
Ritonavir (600 mg bid)	Avoid (↓ etravirine)
Darunavir/ritonavir	No change
Rifabutin, Rifampin	Avoid (↓ etravirine)
Tipranavir/ritonavir	Avoid (↓ etravirine)
Saquinavir/ritonavir	No change

Drug Interactions: Etravirine is a substrate for the liver enzymes CYP3A4, CYP2C9, and CYP2C19. Co-administration with drugs that inhibit or induce these enzymes may alter the therapeutic effect or adverse reaction profile of etravirine or concomitant drug. Amiodarone, bepridil, disopyramide, flecainide, lidocaine (systemic), mexiletine, propafenone, quinidine (↓ antiarrhythmic levels); warfarin (↑ warfarin levels); carbamazepine, phenobarbital, phenytoin (↓ etravirine levels); antifungals (↑ etravirine levels) — also etravirine decreases itraconazole and ketoconazole levels and increases voriconazole levels but has no effect on fluconazole or posaconazole levels; clarithromycin (↑ etravirine levels, ↓ clarithromycin levels), atorvastatin (↓ atorvastatin levels), sildenafil (↓ sildenafil levels), tadalafil (↓ tadalafil levels), vardenafil (↓ vardenafil levels); etravirine has no effect on methadone levels

Adverse Effects: Hypertension, rash, abdominal pain, nausea, diarrhea, ↑ liver enzymes AST(SGOT)/ALT(SGPT), myocardial infarction, hypersensitivity reaction

Allergic Potential: Low (< 2%)

Safety in Pregnancy: B

Comments: Severe and potentially life-threatening skin reactions have been reported, including Stevens-Johnson syndrome, hypersensitivity reaction, and erythema multiforme. Discontinue treatment if severe rash develops. Efficacy in treatment-naive patients has not been established. Take with meals; food increases systemic exposure by 50%

Cerebrospinal Fluid Penetration: No data

REFERENCES:

Lazzarin A, Campbell T, Clotet B, et al. Efficacy and safety of TMC125 (etravirine) in treatment-experienced HIV-1-infected patients in DUET-2: 24-week results from a randomised, double-blind, placebo-controlled trial. Lancet 370:39-48, 2007.

Madruga JV, Cahn P, Grinsztejn B, et al. Efficacy and safety of TMC125 (etravirine) in treatment-experienced HIV-1-infected patients in DUET-1: 24-week results from a randomised, double-blind, placebo-controlled trial. Lancet 370:29-38, 2007.

Production Information: INTELENCE™ oral tablets, etravirine oral tablets. Tibotec Therapeutics, Inc., Raritan, NJ, 2008.

Website: www.intelence-info.com

Fosamprenavir (Lexiva) FPV

Drug Class: Antiretroviral protease inhibitor

Usual Dose: 1400 mg (PO) q12h (without ritonavir); in combination with ritonavir: either 1400 mg (PO) q24h plus ritonavir 200 mg (PO) q24h or 700 mg (PO) q12h plus ritonavir 100 mg (PO) q12h. For PI-experienced patients: 700 mg (PO) q12h plus ritonavir 100 mg (PO) q12h

Pharmacokinetic Parameters:

Peak serum level: 4.8 mcg/mL

Bioavailability: No data

Excreted unchanged (urine) (urine): 1%

Serum half-life (normal/ESRD): 7 hrs/no data

Plasma protein binding: 90%

Volume of distribution (V_d): 6.1 L/kg

Primary Mode of Elimination: Hepatic

Dosage Adjustments*

CrCl 50-80 mL/min	No change
CrCl 10-50 mL/min	No change
CrCl < 10 mL/min	No change
Post–HD or PD dose	No change
CVVH dose	No change
Mild-moderate hepatic insufficiency (Child-Pugh score 5-8)	700 mg (PO) q12h if given without ritonavir; no data with ritonavir
Severe hepatic insufficiency (Child-Pugh score 9-12)	Avoid

Antiretroviral Dosage Adjustments:

Didanosine	Administer didanosine 1 hour apart
Delavirdine	Avoid combination
Efavirenz	Fosamprenavir 700 mg q12h + ritonavir 100 mg q12h + efavirenz; fosamprenavir 1400 mg q24h + ritonavir 200 mg q24h + efavirenz; no data for fosamprenavir 1400 mg q12h + efavirenz
Indinavir	No information
Lopinavir/ritonavir	Avoid
Nelfinavir	No information
Nevirapine	Avoid
Saquinavir	No information
Rifampin	Avoid combination
Rifabutin	Reduce usual rifabutin dose by 50% (or 75% if given with fosamprenavir plus ritonavir; max. 150 mg q48h)

Drug Interactions: Antiretrovirals (see dose adjustment grid, above). Contraindicated with: ergot derivatives, cisapride, midazolam, triazolam, pimozide, (flecainide and propafenone if administered with ritonavir). Do not coadminister with: rifampin, lovastatin, simvastatin, St. John's wort, delavirdine. Dose reduction (of other drug): atorvastatin, rifabutin, sildenafil, vardenafil, ketoconazole, itraconazole. Concentration monitoring (of other drug): amiodarone, systemic lidocaine, quinidine, warfarin (INR), tricyclic antidepressants, cyclosporin, tacrolimus, sirolimus. H_2 blockers and proton pump inhibitors interfere with absorption. Sildenafil (do not give > 25 mg/48 hrs); tadalafil (max. 10 mg/72 hrs); vardenafil (max. 2.5 mg/72 hrs)

Adverse Effects: Rash, Stevens-Johnson syndrome (rare), GI upset, headache, depression, diarrhea, hyperglycemia (including worsening diabetes, new-onset diabetes, DKA), ↑ cholesterol/triglycerides (evaluate risk for coronary disease/pancreatitis), fat redistribution, ↑ SGOT/SGPT, possible increased bleeding in hemophilia

Allergic Potential: High. Fosamprenavir is a sulfonamide; use with caution in patients with sulfonamide allergies

Safety in Pregnancy: C

Comments: Usually given in conjunction with ritonavir. May be taken with or without food. Fosamprenavir is a prodrug that is rapidly hydrolyzed to amprenavir by gut epithelium during absorption. Amprenavir inhibits CYP3A4. Fosamprenavir contains a sulfonamide moiety (as do darunavir and tipranavir)

REFERENCES:

Becker S, Thornton L. Fosamprenavir: advancing HIV protease inhibitor treatment options. Expert Opin Pharmacother 5:1995-2005, 2004.

Chapman TM, Plosker GL, Perry CM. Fosamprenavir: a

"Usual dose" assumes normal renal/hepatic function. * For renal insufficiency, give usual dose x 1 followed by maintenance dose per CrCl. For dialysis patients, dose the same as for CrCl < 10 mL/min and give supplemental (post-HD/PD dose) immediately after dialysis. CrCl = creatinine clearance; CVVH = continuous veno-venous hemofiltration; HD/PD = hemodialysis/peritoneal dialysis. See pp. 147-150 for explanations, p. 3 for abbreviations

review of its use in the management of antiretroviral therapy-naive patients with HIV infection. Drugs 64:2101-24, 2004.
Lexiva (fosamprenavir) approved. AIDS Treat News 31;2, 2003.
Panel on Clinical Practices for Treatment of HIV Infection. Guidelines for the Use of Antiretroviral Agents in HIV-Infected Adults and Adolescents. Department of Health and Human Services. www.aidsinfo.nih.gov/guidelines/. Jan 29, 2008.
Rodriguez-French A, Boghossian J, Gray GE, et al. The NEAT study: a 48-week open-label study to compare the antiviral efficacy and safety of GW433908 versus nelfinavir in antiretroviral therapy-naive HIV-1-infected patients. J Acquir Immune Defic Syndr 35: 22-32, 2004.
Website: www.TreatHIV.com

Indinavir (Crixivan) IDV

Drug Class: Antiretroviral protease inhibitor
Usual Dose: 800 mg (PO) q8h
Pharmacokinetic Parameters:
Peak serum level: 252 mcg/mL
Bioavailability: 65% (77% with food)
Excreted unchanged (urine): < 20%
Serum half-life (normal/ESRD): 2 hrs/no data
Plasma protein binding: 60 %
Volume of distribution (V_d): No data
Primary Mode of Elimination: Hepatic
Dosage Adjustments*

CrCl 50–80 mL/min	No change
CrCl 10–50 mL/min	No change
CrCl < 10 mL/min	No change
Post–HD dose	None
Post–PD dose	None
CVVH dose	No change
Moderate hepatic insufficiency	600 mg (PO) q8h
Severe hepatic insufficiency	400 mg (PO) q8h

Antiretroviral Dosage Adjustments:

Didanosine	Administer didanosine 1 hour apart
Delavirdine	Indinavir 600 mg q8h
Efavirenz	Indinavir 1000 mg q8h
Lopinavir/ritonavir	Indinavir 600 mg q12h
Nelfinavir	Limited data for indinavir 1200 mg q12h + nelfinavir 1250 mg q12h
Nevirapine	Indinavir 1000 mg q8h
Ritonavir	Indinavir 800 mg q12h + ritonavir 100-200 mg q12h, or 400 mg q12h of each drug
Saquinavir	No information
Rifampin	Avoid combination
Rifabutin	Indinavir 1000 mg q8h; rifabutin 150 mg q24h or 300 mg 2-3x/week

Drug Interactions: Antiretrovirals, rifabutin, rifampin (see dose adjustment grid, above); astemizole, terfenadine, benzodiazepines, cisapride, ergot alkaloids, statins, St. John's wort (avoid if possible); calcium channel blockers (↑ calcium channel blocker levels); carbamazepine, phenobarbital, phenytoin (↓ indinavir levels, ↑ anticonvulsant levels; monitor); tenofovir (↓ indinavir levels, ↑ tenofovir levels); clarithromycin, erythromycin, telithromycin (↑ indinavir and macrolide levels); didanosine (administer indinavir on empty stomach 1 hour apart); ethinyl estradiol, norethindrone (↑ interacting drug levels; no dosage adjustment); grapefruit juice (↓ indinavir levels); itraconazole, ketoconazole (↑ indinavir levels); sildenafil (↑ or ↓ sildenafil levels; do not exceed 25 mg in 48

"Usual dose" assumes normal renal/hepatic function. * For renal insufficiency, give usual dose x 1 followed by maintenance dose per CrCl. For dialysis patients, dose the same as for CrCl < 10 mL/min and give supplemental (post-HD/PD dose) immediately after dialysis. CrCl = creatinine clearance; CVVH = continuous veno-venous hemofiltration; HD/PD = hemodialysis/peritoneal dialysis. See pp. 147-150 for explanations, p. 3 for abbreviations

hrs), tadalafil (max. 10 mg/72 hrs), vardenafil (max 2.5 mg/72 hrs); theophylline (↓ theophylline levels); fluticasone nasal spray (avoid concomitant use)

Adverse Effects: Nephrolithiasis, nausea, vomiting, diarrhea, anemia, leukopenia, headache, insomnia, hyperglycemia (including worsening diabetes, new-onset diabetes, DKA), ↑ SGOT/SGPT, ↑ indirect bilirubin (2° to drug-induced Gilbert's syndrome; inconsequential), fat redistribution, lipid abnormalities (evaluate risk of coronary disease/pancreatitis), abdominal pain, possible ↑ bleeding in hemophilia, dry skin, chelitis, paronychiae

Allergic Potential: Low

Safety in Pregnancy: C

Comments: Renal stone formation may be prevented/minimized by adequate hydration (1-3 liters water daily); ↑ risk of nephrolithiasis with alcohol. Take 1 hour before or 2 hours after meals (may take with skim milk or low fat meal). Separate dosing with ddI by 1 hour.

Cerebrospinal Fluid Penetration: 16%

REFERENCES:

Acosta EP, Henry K, Baken L, et al. Indinavir concentrations and antiviral effect. Pharmacotherapy 19:708-712, 1999.

Antinori A, Giancola MI, Griserri S, et al. Factors influencing virological response to antiretroviral drugs in cerebrospinal fluid of advanced HIV-1-infected patients. AIDS 16:1867-76, 2002.

Deeks SG, Smith M, Holodniy M, et al. HIV-1 protease inhibitors: A review for clinicians. JAMA 277:145-53, 1997.

DiCenzo R, Forrest A, Fischl MA, et al. Pharmacokinetics of indinavir and nelfinavir in treatment-naive, human immunodeficiency virus-infected subjects. Antimicrob Agents Chemother 48:918-23, 2004.

Go J, Cunha BA. Indinavir: A review. Antibiotics for Clinicians 3:81-87, 1999.

Justesen US, Andersen AB, Klitgaard NA, et al. Pharmacokinetic interaction between rifampin and the combination of indinavir and low-dose ritonavir in HIV-infected patients. Clin Infect Dis 38:426-9, 2004.

Kopp JB, Falloon J, Filie A, et al. Indinavir-associated intestinal nephritis and urothelial inflammation: clinical and cytologic findings. Clin Infect Dis 34:1122-8, 2002.

Meraviglia P, Angeli E, Del Sorbo F, et al. Risk factors for indinavir-related renal colic in HIV patients: predicative value of indinavir dose-body mass index. AIDS 16:2089-2093, 2002.

McDonald CK, Kuritzkes DR. Human immunodeficiency virus type 1 protease inhibitors. Arch Intern Med 157:951-9, 1997.

Panel on Clinical Practices for Treatment of HIV Infection. Guidelines for the use of antiretroviral agents in HIV-infected adults and adolescents. Department of Health and Human Services. www.aidsinfo.nih.gov/guidelines/. Jan 29, 2008.

Website: www.crixivan.com

Lamivudine (Epivir) 3TC

Drug Class: Antiretroviral NRTI (nucleoside reverse transcriptase inhibitor); antiviral (HBV)

Usual Dose: 150 mg (PO) q12h or 300 mg (PO) q24h (HIV); 100 mg (PO) q24h (HBV)

Pharmacokinetic Parameters:

Peak serum level: 1.5 mcg/mL

Bioavailability: 86%

Excreted unchanged (urine): 71%

Serum half-life (normal/ESRD): 5-7/20 hrs

Plasma protein binding: 36%

Volume of distribution (V_d): 1.3 L/kg

Primary Mode of Elimination: Renal

Dosage Adjustments*

CrCl 30–50 mL/min	150 mg (PO) q24h
CrCl 15–30 mL/min	100 mg (PO) q24h
CrCl 5–15 mL/min	50 mg (PO) q24h
CrCl < 5 mL/min	25 mg (PO) q24h
Post–HD dose	No information
Post–PD dose	No information
CVVH dose	No information
Moderate hepatic insufficiency	No change
Severe hepatic insufficiency	No information

Drug Interactions: Didanosine, zalcitabine (↑ risk of pancreatitis); TMP-SMX (↑ lamivudine levels); zidovudine (↑ zidovudine levels)

Adverse Effects: Drug fever/rash, abdominal pain/diarrhea, nausea, vomiting, anemia, leukopenia, photophobia, depression, cough,

nasal complaints, headache, dizziness, peripheral neuropathy, pancreatitis, myalgias, lactic acidosis with hepatic steatosis (rare, but potentially life-threatening toxicity with NRTI's)
Allergic Potential: Low
Safety in Pregnancy: C
Comments: Potential cross resistance with didanosine. Prevents development of AZT resistance and restores AZT susceptibility. May be taken with or without food. Effective against HBV, but HBV may reactivate after lamivudine therapy is stopped. Also a component of Combivir, Trizivir, and Epzicom.
Cerebrospinal Fluid Penetration: 15%

REFERENCES:

Benson CA, van der Horst C, Lamarca A, et al. A randomized study of emtricitabine and lamivudine in stable suppressed patients with HIV. AIDS 18:2269-2276, 2004.
Eron JJ, Benoit SL, Jemsek J, et al. Treatment with lamivudine, zidovudine, or both in HIV-positive patients with 200 to 500 CD4 cells per cubic millimeter. N Engl J Med 333:1662-9, 1995.
Lai Cl, Chien RN. Leung NW, et al. A one-year trial of lamivudine for chronic hepatitis B. N Engl J Med 339:61-8, 1998.
Lau GK, He ML, Fong DY, et al. Preemptive use of lamivudine reduces hepatitis B exacerbation after allogeneic hematopoietic cell transplantation. Hepatology 36:702-9, 2002.
Leung N. Lamivudine for chronic hepatitis B. Expert Rev Anti Infect Ther 2:173-80, 2004.
Liaw YF, Sung JY, Chow WC, et al. Lamivudine for patients with chronic hepatitis B and advanced liver disease. N Engl J Med 351:1521-31, 2004.
Lu Y, Wang B, Yu L, et al. Lamivudine in prevention and treatment of recurrent HBV after liver transplantation. Hepatobiliary Pancreat Dis Int 3:504-7, 2004.
Marrone A, Zampino R, D'Onofrio M, et al. Combined interferon plus lamivudine treatment in young patients with dual HBV (HbeAg positive) and HCV chronic infection. J Hepatol 41:1064-5, 2004.
Murphy RL, Brun S, Hicks C, et al. ABT-378/ritonavir plus stavudine and lamivudine for the treatment of antiretroviral-naive adults with HIV-1 infection: 48-week results. AIDS 15:F1-9, 2001.
Panel on Clinical Practices for Treatment of HIV Infection. Guidelines for the use of antiretroviral agents in HIV-infected adults and adolescents. Department of Health and Human Services. www.aidsinfo.nih.gov/guidelines/. Jan 29, 2008.
Perry CM, Faulds D. Lamivudine. A review of its antiviral activity, pharmacokinetic properties and therapeutic efficacy in the management of HIV infection. Drugs 53:657-80, 1997.
Rivkina A, Rybalov S. Chronic hepatitis B: current and future treatment options. Pharmacotherapy 22:721-37, 2002.
Schmilovitz-Weiss H, Ben-Ari Z, Sikuler E, et al. Lamivudine treatment for acute severe hepatitis B: a pilot study. Liver Int 24:547-51, 2004.
Staszewski S, Morales-Ramirez J, Trashima KT, et al. Efavirenz plus zidovudine and lamivudine, efavirenz plus indinavir, and indinavir plus zidovudine and lamivudine in the treatment of HIV-1 infection in adults. N Engl J Med 341:1865-1873, 1999.
Website: www.TreatHIV.com

Lamivudine + Zidovudine (Combivir)

Drug Class: Antiretroviral NRTI's combination
Usual Dose: Combivir tablet = 150 mg lamivudine + 300 mg zidovudine. Usual dose = 1 tablet (PO) q12h
Pharmacokinetic Parameters:
Peak serum level: 2.6/1.2 mcg/mL
Bioavailability: 82/60%
Excreted unchanged (urine): 86/64%
Serum half-life (normal/ESRD): [6/1.1]/[20/2.2] hrs
Plasma protein binding: <36/<38%
Volume of distribution (V_d): 1.3/1.6 L/kg
Primary Mode of Elimination: Renal
Dosage Adjustments*

CrCl 50–80 mL/min	No change
CrCl 10–50 mL/min	Avoid
CrCl < 10 mL/min	Avoid
Post–HD dose	Avoid
Post–PD dose	Avoid
CVVH dose	Avoid
Moderate hepatic insufficiency	Avoid
Severe hepatic insufficiency	Avoid

"Usual dose" assumes normal renal/hepatic function. * For renal insufficiency, give usual dose x 1 followed by maintenance dose per CrCl. For dialysis patients, dose the same as for CrCl < 10 mL/min and give supplemental (post-HD/PD dose) immediately after dialysis. CrCl = creatinine clearance; CVVH = continuous veno-venous hemofiltration; HD/PD = hemodialysis/peritoneal dialysis. See pp. 147-150 for explanations, p. 3 for abbreviations

Drug Interactions: Atovaquone (↑ zidovudine levels); stavudine (antagonist to stavudine; avoid combination); ganciclovir, doxorubicin (neutropenia); tipranavir (↓ zidovudine levels); TMP-SMX (↑ lamivudine and zidovudine levels); vinca alkaloids (neutropenia)
Adverse Effects: Most common (>5%): nausea, vomiting, diarrhea, anorexia, insomnia, fever/chills, headache, malaise/fatigue. Others (less common): peripheral neuropathy, myopathy, steatosis, pancreatitis. Lab abnormalities: mild hyperglycemia, anemia, LFT elevations, hypertriglyceridemia, leukopenia
Allergic Potential: Low
Safety in Pregnancy: C
Cerebrospinal Fluid Penetration: Lamivudine = 12%; zidovudine = 60%

REFERENCES:

Drugs for AIDS and associated infections. Med Lett Drug Ther 35:79-86, 1993.
Hirsch MS, D'Aquila RT. Therapy for human immunodeficiency virus infection. N Engl J Med 328:1685-95, 1993.
McLeod GX, Hammer SM. Zidovudine: Five years later. Ann Intern Med 117:487-510, 1992.
Panel on Clinical Practices for Treatment of HIV Infection. Guidelines for the use of antiretroviral agents in HIV-infected adults and adolescents. Department of Health and Human Services. www.aidsinfo.nih.gov/guidelines/. Jan 29, 2008.
Staszewski S, Morales-Ramirez J, Trashima KT, et al. Efavirenz plus zidovudine and lamivudine, efavirenz plus indinavir, and indinavir plus zidovudine and lamivudine in the treatment of HIV-1 infection in adults. N Engl J Med 341:1865-1873, 1999.
Website: www.TreatHIV.com

Lopinavir + Ritonavir (Kaletra) LPV/r

Drug Class: Antiretroviral protease inhibitor combination
Usual Dose: Therapy-naive: 400/10 mg (2 tablets or 5 mL solution) q12h or 800/200 mg (4 tablets or 10 mL solution) q24h. Therapy-experienced: 400/100 mg q12h. New tablet formulation (lopinavir 200 mg + ritonavir 50 mg) replaces capsules (lopinavir 133.3 mg + ritonavir 33.3 mg), resulting in reduction in total number of pills from 6 capsules to 4 tablets per day. Also available as an oral solution (lopinavir 400 mg + ritonavir 100 mg per 5 mL)
Pharmacokinetic Parameters:
Peak serum level: 9.6/≤ 1 mcg/mL
Bioavailability: No data
Excreted unchanged (urine): 3%
Serum half-life (normal/ESRD): 5-6/5-6 hrs
Plasma protein binding: 99%
Volume of distribution (V_d): No data/ 0.44 L/kg
Primary Mode of Elimination: Hepatic
Dosage Adjustments*

CrCl 50–80 mL/min	No change
CrCl 10–50 mL/min	No change
CrCl < 10 mL/min	No change
Post–HD dose	None
Post–PD dose	None
CVVH dose	No change
Moderate hepatic insufficiency	No change
Severe hepatic insufficiency	Avoid

Antiretroviral Dosage Adjustments:

Fosamprenavir	Avoid
Delavirdine	No information
Efavirenz	Consider lopinavir/ritonavir 600/150 mg (3 tablets) q12h
Indinavir	Indinavir 600 mg q12h
Nelfinavir	Same as for efavirenz
Nevirapine	Same as for efavirenz
Rifabutin	Max. dose of rifabutin 150 mg qod or 3 times per week

"Usual dose" assumes normal renal/hepatic function. * For renal insufficiency, give usual dose x 1 followed by maintenance dose per CrCl. For dialysis patients, dose the same as for CrCl < 10 mL/min and give supplemental (post-HD/PD dose) immediately after dialysis. CrCl = creatinine clearance; CVVH = continuous veno-venous hemofiltration; HD/PD = hemodialysis/peritoneal dialysis. See pp. 147-150 for explanations, p. 3 for abbreviations

Saquinavir	Saquinavir 1000 mg q12h

Drug Interactions: Antiretrovirals, rifabutin, (see dose adjustment grid, above); astemizole, terfenadine, benzodiazepines, cisapride, ergotamine, flecainide, pimozide, propafenone, rifampin, statins, St. John's wort (avoid if possible); tenofovir (↓ lopinavir levels, ↑ tenofovir levels). ↓ effectiveness of oral contraceptives. Insufficient data on other drug interactions listed for ritonavir alone

Adverse Effects: Diarrhea (very common), headache, nausea, vomiting, asthenia, ↑ SGOT/SGPT, hepatotoxicity, abdominal pain, pancreatitis, paresthesias, hyperglycemia (including worsening diabetes, new-onset diabetes, DKA), ↑ cholesterol/triglycerides (evaluate risk for coronary disease, pancreatitis), ↑ CPK, ↑ uric acid, fat redistribution, possible increased bleeding in hemophilia. Oral solution contains 42.4% alcohol

Allergic Potential: Low

Safety in Pregnancy: C

Comments: New tablet formulation does not require refrigeration and may be taken with or without food. With oral solution, Lopinavir serum concentrations with moderately fatty meals are increased 54%

REFERENCES:

Benson CA, Deeks SG, Brun SC, et al. Safety and antiviral activity at 48 weeks of lopinavir/ritonavir plus nevirapine and 2 nucleoside reverse-transcriptase inhibitors in human immunodeficiency virus type 1-infected protease inhibitor-experienced patients. J Infect Dis 185:599-607, 2002.

Fischl MA. Antiretroviral therapy in 1999 for antiretroviral-naive individuals with HIV infection. AIDS 13:49-59, 1999.

Manfredi R, Calza L, Chiodo F. First-line efavirenz versus lopinavir-ritonavir-based highly active antiretroviral therapy for naive patients. AIDS 18:2331-2333, 2004.

Panel on Clinical Practices for Treatment of HIV Infection. Guidelines for the use of antiretroviral agents in HIV-infected adults and adolescents. Department of Health and Human Services. www.aidsinfo.nih.gov/guidelines/. Jan 29, 2008.

Walmsley S, Bernstein B, King M, et al. Lopinavir-ritonavir versus nelfinavir for the initial treatment of HIV infection. N Engl J Med 346:2039-46, 2002.

Website: www.kaletra.com

Maraviroc (Selzentry) MVC

Drug Class: HIV-1 chemokine receptor 5 (CCR5) antagonist

Usual Dose: 150 mg, 300 mg, or 600 mg (PO) q12h, depending on concomitant medications (see below), in CCR5-tropic HIV-1 isolates. Available in 150 mg and 300 mg tablets

Pharmacokinetic Parameters:

Peak serum level: 266-618 mcg/mL

Bioavailability: 23-33%

Excreted unchanged: 20% (urine); 76% (feces)

Serum half-life (normal/ESRD): 14-18 hrs/not studied

Plasma protein binding: 76%

Volume of distribution (V_d): 194 L

Primary Mode of Elimination: Fecal/renal

Dosage Adjustments*

CrCl 50–80 mL/min	No change
CrCl 10–25 mL/min	Use caution
CrCl < 10 mL/min	Use caution
Post–HD dose	No information
Post–PD dose	No information
CVVH dose	No information
Mild hepatic insufficiency	No information
Moderate or severe hepatic insufficiency	No information

Antiretroviral Dosage Adjustments:

protease inhibitors (except tipranavir/ritonavir), delavirdine, ketoconazole, itraconazole, clarithromycin, nefazodone, telithromycin	150 mg (PO) q12h

"Usual dose" assumes normal renal/hepatic function. * For renal insufficiency, give usual dose x 1 followed by maintenance dose per CrCl. For dialysis patients, dose the same as for CrCl < 10 mL/min and give supplemental (post-HD/PD dose) immediately after dialysis. CrCl = creatinine clearance; CVVH = continuous veno-venous hemofiltration; HD/PD = hemodialysis/peritoneal dialysis. See pp. 147-150 for explanations, p. 3 for abbreviations

tipranavir/ritonavir, nevirapine, all NRTIs and enfuvirtide	300 mg (PO) q12h
efavirenz, rifampin, carbamazepine, phenobarbital, phenytoin	600 mg (PO) q12h

Drug Interactions: Maraviroc is a substrate of CYP3A and P-glycoprotein and is likely to be modulated by inhibitors and inducers of these enzymes/transporters

Adverse Effects: Hepatotoxicity has been reported. A systemic allergic reaction (e.g., pruritic rash, eosinophilia, or elevated IgE) prior to the development of hepatotoxicity may occur. Other adverse effects: cough, infection, upper respiratory tract infection, rash, pyrexia, dizziness, abdominal pain, musculoskeletal symptoms (joint/muscle pain). Myocardial infarction/ischemia reported in < 2% in clinical trials

Allergic Potential: Low

Safety in Pregnancy: B

Comments: Indicated for treatment-experienced adult patients infected with only cellular chemokine receptor (CCR) 5–tropic HIV-1 virus detectable who have evidence of viral replication and HIV-1 strains resistant to multiple antiretroviral agents. Used in combination with other antiretroviral agents. Trofile phenotype test (performed at Monogram) is needed to confirm infection with CCR5-tropic HIV-1 (also known as "R5 virus")

Cerebrospinal Fluid Penetration: No data

REFERENCES:

Dorr P, Westby M, Dobbs S, et al. Maraviroc (UK-427,857), a potent, orally bioavailable, and selective small-molecule inhibitor of chemokine receptor CCR5 with broad-spectrum anti-human immunodeficiency virus type 1 activity. Antimicrob Agents Chemother 49:4721-4732, 2005.

Lalezari, J. Efficacy and Safety of Maraviroc plus Optimized Background Therapy in Viremic ART-experienced Patients Infected with CCR5-tropic HIV-1: 24-Week Results of a Phase 2b/3 Study in the US and Canada [Abstract 104bLB]. Conference on Retroviruses and Opportunistic Infections. Alexandria, VA. 2007. Available from URL: http://www.retroconference.org/2007/Abstracts/30635.htm

Lederman MM, Penn-Nicholson A, Cho M, et al. Biology of CCR5 and its role in HIV infection and treatment. JAMA 296:815-826, 2006.

Nelson, M. Efficacy and Safety of Maraviroc plus Optimized Background Therapy in Viremic, ART-experienced Patients Infected with CCR5-tropic HIV-1 in Europe, Australia, and North America: 24-Week Results [Abstract 104aLB]. Conference on Retroviruses and Opportunistic Infections. Alexandria, VA. 2007. Available from URL: http://www.retroconference.org/2007/Abstracts/30636.htm

Product Information: SELZENTRY(R) oral tablets, maraviroc oral tablets. Pfizer Labs, New York, NY, 2007.

US Department of Health and Human Services Panel on Antiretroviral Therapy Guidelines for Adults and Adolescents: DHHS Perinatal Panel notice on nelfinavir FDA-Pfizer letter. US Department of Health and Human Services. Washington, DC. 2007. Available from URL: http://aidsinfo.nih.gov/contentfiles/PeriNFVNotice.pdf

Website: www.selzentry.com

Nelfinavir (Viracept) NFV

Drug Class: Antiretroviral protease inhibitor

Usual Dose: 1250 mg (PO) q12h (two 625-mg tablets per dose) with meals, or five 250-mg tabs or 750 mg (three 250-mg tabs) (PO) q8h

Pharmacokinetic Parameters:

Peak serum level: 35 mcg/mL

Bioavailability: 20-80%

Excreted unchanged (urine): 1-2%

Serum half-life (normal/ESRD): 4 hrs/no data

Plasma protein binding: 98%

Volume of distribution (V_d): 5 L/kg

Primary Mode of Elimination: Hepatic

Dosage Adjustments*

CrCl 50–80 mL/min	No change
CrCl 10–50 mL/min	No change
CrCl < 10 mL/min	No change
Post–HD dose	None
Post-PD dose	None
CVVH dose	No change

"Usual dose" assumes normal renal/hepatic function. * For renal insufficiency, give usual dose x 1 followed by maintenance dose per CrCl. For dialysis patients, dose the same as for CrCl < 10 mL/min and give supplemental (post-HD/PD dose) immediately after dialysis. CrCl = creatinine clearance; CVVH = continuous veno-venous hemofiltration; HD/PD = hemodialysis/peritoneal dialysis. See pp. 147-150 for explanations, p. 3 for abbreviations

Moderate hepatic insufficiency	No information
Severe hepatic insufficiency	No information – use caution

Antiretroviral Dosage Adjustments:

Delavirdine	No information (monitor for neutropenia)
Efavirenz	No changes
Indinavir	Limited data for nelfinavir 1250 mg q12h + indinavir 1200 mg q12h
Lopinavir/ritonavir	Nelfinavir 1000 mg q12h or lopinavir/r 600/150 mg q12h
Nevirapine	No information
Ritonavir	No information
Saquinavir	Saquinavir 1200 mg q12h
Rifampin	Avoid combination
Rifabutin	Nelfinavir 1250 mg q12h; rifabutin 150 mg q24h or 300 mg 2-3x/week

Drug Interactions: Antiretrovirals, rifabutin, rifampin (see dose adjustment grid, above); amiodarone, quinidine, astemizole, terfenadine, benzodiazepines, cisapride, ergot alkaloids, statins, St. John's wort (avoid if possible); carbamazepine, phenytoin, phenobarbital (↓ nelfinavir levels, ↑ anticonvulsant levels; monitor); caspofungin (↓ caspofungin levels, may ↓ caspofungin effect); clarithromycin, erythromycin, telithromycin (↑ nelfinavir and macrolide levels); didanosine (dosing conflict with food; give nelfinavir with food 2 hours before or 1 hour after didanosine); itraconazole, voriconazole, ketoconazole (↑ nelfinavir levels); lamivudine (↑ lamivudine levels); methadone (may require ↑ methadone dose); oral contraceptives, zidovudine (↓ zidovudine levels); sildenafil (↑ or ↓ sildenafil levels; do not exceed 25 mg in 48 hrs, tadalafil (max. 10 mg/72 hrs, vardenafil (max. 2.5 mg/72 hrs)

Adverse Effects: Impaired concentration, nausea, abdominal pain, secretory diarrhea, ↑ SGOT/SGPT, rash, ↑ cholesterol/triglycerides (evaluate risk for coronary disease/pancreatitis), fat redistribution, hyperglycemia (including worsening diabetes, new-onset diabetes, DKA), possible increased bleeding in hemophilia

Allergic Potential: Low

Safety in Pregnancy: B

Comments: Take with food (absorption increased 300%). New 625-mg tablet available

Cerebrospinal Fluid Penetration: Undetectable

REFERENCES:

Albrecht MA, Bosch RJ, Hammer SM, et al. Nelfinavir, efavirenz, or both after the failure of nucleoside treatment of HIV infection. N Engl J Med 345:398-407, 2001.

Clotet B, Ruiz L, Martinez-Picado J, et al. Prevalence of HIV protease mutations on failure of nelfinavir-containing HAART: a retrospective analysis of four clinical studies and two observational cohorts. HIV Clin Trials 3:316-23, 2002.

Deeks SG, Smith M, Holodniy M, et al. HIV-1 protease inhibitors: A review for clinicians. JAMA 277:145-53, 1997.

DiCenzo R, Forrest A, Fischl MA, et al. Pharmacokinetics of indinavir and nelfinavir in treatment-naive, human immunodeficiency virus-infected subjects. Antimicrob Agents Chemother 48:918-23, 2004.

Go J, Cunha BA. Nelfinavir: A review. Antibiotics for Clinicians 4:17-23, 2000.

Kaul DR, Cinti SK, Carver PL, et al. HIV protease inhibitors: Advances in therapy and adverse reactions, including metabolic complications. Pharmacotherapy 19:281-98, 1999.

Panel on Clinical Practices for Treatment of HIV Infection. Guidelines for the use of antiretroviral agents in HIV-infected adults and adolescents. Department of Health and Human Services. www.aidsinfo.nih.gov/guidelines/. Jan 29, 2008.

Perry CM, Benfield P. Nelfinavir. Drugs 54:81-7, 1997.

Simpson KN, Luo MP, Chumney E, et al. Cost-effective of lopinavir/ritonavir versus nelfinavir as the first-line highly active antiretroviral therapy regimen for HIV infection. HIV Clin Trials 5:294-304, 2004.

Walmsley S, Bernstein B, King M, et al. Lopinavir-

ritonavir versus nelfinavir for the initial treatment of HIV infection. N Engl J Med 346:2039-46, 2002.
Website: www.viracept.com

Nevirapine (Viramune) NVP

Drug Class: Antiretroviral NNRTI (non-nucleoside reverse transcriptase inhibitor)
Usual Dose: 200 mg (PO) q24h x 2 weeks, then 200 mg (PO) q12h
Pharmacokinetic Parameters:
Peak serum level: 0.9-3.6 mcg/mL
Bioavailability: 90%
Excreted unchanged (urine): 5%
Serum half-life (normal/ESRD): 40 hrs/no data
Plasma protein binding: 60%
Volume of distribution (V_d): 1.4 L/kg
Primary Mode of Elimination: Hepatic
Dosage Adjustments*

CrCl 50–80 mL/min	No change
CrCl 10–50 mL/min	No change
CrCl < 20 mL/min	No change; use caution
Post–HD dose	200 mg (PO)
Post–PD dose	None
CVVH dose	No change
Moderate hepatic insufficiency	Use caution
Severe hepatic insufficiency	Avoid

Antiretroviral Dosage Adjustments:

Delavirdine	No information
Efavirenz	No information
Indinavir	Indinavir 1000 mg q8h
Lopinavir/ritonavir (l/r)	Consider l/r 600/150 mg q12h in PI-experienced patients
Nelfinavir	No information
Ritonavir	No changes
Saquinavir	No information
Rifampin	Not recommended
Rifabutin	Use caution

Drug Interactions: Antiretrovirals, rifabutin, rifampin (see dose adjustment grid, above); carbamazepine, phenobarbital, phenytoin (monitor anticonvulsant levels); caspofungin (↓ caspofungin levels, may ↓ caspofungin effect); ethinyl estradiol (↓ ethinyl estradiol levels; use additional/alternative method); ketoconazole (avoid); voriconazole (↑ nevirapine levels); methadone (↓ methadone levels; titrate methadone dose to effect); tacrolimus (↓ tacrolimus levels)
Adverse Effects: Drug fever/rash (may be severe; usually occurs within 6 weeks), Stevens–Johnson syndrome, ↑ SGOT/SGPT, ***fatal hepatitis***, headache, diarrhea, leukopenia, stomatitis, peripheral neuropathy, paresthesias. Greater risk of fatal hepatitis and Stevens-Johnson syndrome when CD4 > 400/mm^3 (males) or > 250/mm^3 (females) (monitor patients intensely for first 18 weeks of therapy)
Allergic Potential: High
Safety in Pregnancy: C
Comments: Absorption not affected by food. Not to be used for post-exposure prophylaxis because of potential for fatal hepatitis.
Cerebrospinal Fluid Penetration: 45%

REFERENCES:

D'Aquila RT, Hughes MD, Johnson VA, et al. Nevirapine, zidovudine, and didanosine compared with zidovudine and didanosine in patients with HIV-1 infection. Ann Intern Med 124:1019-30, 1996.
Hammer SM, Kessler HA, Saag MS. Issues in combination antiretroviral therapy: A review. J Acquired Immune Defic Syndr 7:24-37, 1994.
Havlir DV. Lange JM. New antiretrovirals and new combinations. AIDS 12:165-74, 1998.
Herzmann C, Karcher H. Nevirapine plus zidovudine to prevent mother-to-child transmission of HIV. N Engl J Med 351:2013-5, 2004.
Johnson S, Chan J, Bennett CL. Hepatotoxicity after prophylaxis with a nevirapine-containing antiretroviral regimen. Ann Intern Med 137:146-7, 2002.
Milinkovic A, Martinez E. Nevirapine in the treatment of

"Usual dose" assumes normal renal/hepatic function. * For renal insufficiency, give usual dose x 1 followed by maintenance dose per CrCl. For dialysis patients, dose the same as for CrCl < 10 mL/min and give supplemental (post-HD/PD dose) immediately after dialysis. CrCl = creatinine clearance; CVVH = continuous veno-venous hemofiltration; HD/PD = hemodialysis/peritoneal dialysis. See pp. 147-150 for explanations, p. 3 for abbreviations

HIV. Expert Rev Anti Infect Ther 2:367-73, 2004.
Montaner JS, Reiss P, Cooper D, et al. A randomized, double-blind trial comparing combinations of nevirapine, didanosine, and zidovudine for HIV-infected patients: The INCAS trial. Italy, the Netherlands, Canada and Australia Study. J Am Med Assoc 279:930-937, 1998.
Negredo E, Ribalta J, Paredes R, et al. Reversal of atherogenic lipoprotein profile in HIV-1 infected patients with lipodystrophy after replacing protease inhibitors by nevirapine. AIDS 16:1383-9, 2002.
Panel on Clinical Practices for Treatment of HIV Infection. Guidelines for the use of antiretroviral agents in HIV-infected adults and adolescents. Department of Health and Human Services. www.aidsinfo.nih.gov/guidelines/. Jan 29, 2008.
Weverling GJ, Lange JM, Jurriaans S, et al. Alternative multidrug regimen provides improved suppression of HIV-1 replication over triple therapy. AIDS 12:117-22, 1998.
Website: www.viramune.com

Raltegravir (Isentress) RAL

Drug Class: HIV-1 integrase inhibitor
Usual Dose: 400 mg (PO) q12h
Pharmacokinetic Parameters:
Peak serum level: 6.5 μM
Bioavailability: ~ 32% (20%-43%)
Excreted unchanged: 51% (feces); 9% (urine)
Serum half-life (normal/ESRD): 9-12 hrs/no data
Plasma protein binding: 83 %
Volume of distribution (Vd): not studied
Primary Mode of Elimination: Fecal/renal
Dosage Adjustments*

CrCl 50–80 mL/min	No change
CrCl 10–50 mL/min	No change
CrCl < 10 mL/min	No information
Post–HD dose	No information
Post–PD dose	No information
CVVH dose	No information
Mild/moderate hepatic insufficiency	No change
Severe hepatic insufficiency	No information

Antiretroviral Dosage Adjustments:

Atazanavir	No change
Atazanavir/ritonavir	No change
Efavirenz	No change
Rifampin	Avoid
Ritonavir	No change
Tenofovir	No change
Tipranavir/ritonavir	No change

Drug Interactions: Rifampin (↓ raltegravir levels, use with caution). In-vitro, raltegravir does not inhibit CYP1A2, CYP2B6, CYP2C8, CYP2C9, CYP2C19, CYP2D6 or CYP3A and does not induce CYP3A4. In addition, raltegravir does not inhibit P-glycoprotein-mediated transport. Raltegravir is therefore not expected to affect the pharmacokinetics of drugs that are substrates of these enzymes or P-glycoprotein (e.g., protease inhibitors, NNRTIs, methadone, opioid analgesics, statins, azole antifungals, proton pump inhibitors, oral contraceptives, anti-erectile dysfunction agents)
Adverse Effects: Nausea, headache, diarrhea, pyrexia
Allergic Potential: Low
Safety in Pregnancy: C
Comments: May be taken with or without food. CPK elevations, myopathy and rhabdomyolysis have been reported — use with caution in patients at increased risk for myopathy or rhabdomyolysis, such as those receiving concomitant medications known to cause these conditions (e.g., statins). Raltegravir is indicated for treatment-experienced adult patients who have evidence of viral replication and HIV-1 strains resistant to multiple antiretroviral agents
Cerebrospinal Fluid Penetration: No data

REFERENCES:

Cooper D, et al. CROI 2008. Feb, 2008. Boston, MA. Abstr 788.
Grinsztejn B, Nguyen BY, Katlama C, et al. Safety and efficacy of the HIV-1 integrase inhibitor raltegravir (MK-0518) in treatment-experienced patients with

"Usual dose" assumes normal renal/hepatic function. * For renal insufficiency, give usual dose x 1 followed by maintenance dose per CrCl. For dialysis patients, dose the same as for CrCl < 10 mL/min and give supplemental (post-HD/PD dose) immediately after dialysis. CrCl = creatinine clearance; CVVH = continuous veno-venous hemofiltration; HD/PD = hemodialysis/peritoneal dialysis. See pp. 147-150 for explanations, p. 3 for abbreviations

multidrug-resistant virus: a phase II randomised controlled trial. Lancet 369:1261-1269, 2007.
Iwamoto M, Wenning LA, Petry AS, et al. Safety, tolerability, and pharmacokinetics of raltegravir after single and multiple doses in healthy subjects. Clin Pharmacol Ther 2007.
Kassahun K, McIntosh I, Cui D, et al. Metabolism and Disposition in Humans of Raltegravir (MK-0518), an Anti-AIDS Drug Targeting the HIV-1 Integrase Enzyme. Drug Metab Dispos Epub:1-28, 2007.
Markowitz M, Morales-Ramirez JO, Nguyen BY, et al. Antiretroviral activity, pharmacokinetics, and tolerability of MK-0518, a novel inhibitor of HIV-1 integrase, dosed as monotherapy for 10 days in treatment-naive HIV-1-infected individuals. J Acquir Immune Defic Syndr 43:509-515, 2006.
Palmisano L. Role of integrase inhibitors in the treatment of HIV disease. Expert Rev Anti Infect Ther 5:67-75, 2007.
Product Information. ISENTRESS oral tablets, raltegravir oral tablets. Merck & Co,Inc, Whitehouse Station, NJ, 2007.
Steigbigel, R. Results of BENCHMRK-2, a Phase III Study Evaluating the Efficacy and Safety of MK-0518, a Novel HIV-1 Integrase Inhibitor, in Patients with Triple-class Resistant Virus [Abstract 105bLB]. Conference on Retroviruses and Opportunistic Infections. Alexandria, VA. 2007. Available from URL: http://www.retroconference.org/2007/Abstracts/30688.htm
Website: www.isentress.com

Ritonavir (Norvir) RTV

Drug Class: Antiretroviral protease inhibitor
Usual Dose: 600 mg (PO) q12h (see comments)
Pharmacokinetic Parameters:
Peak serum level: 11 mcg/mL
Bioavailability: No data
Excreted unchanged (urine): 3.5%
Serum half-life (normal/ESRD): 4 hrs/no data
Plasma protein binding: 99%
Volume of distribution (V_d): 0.41 L/kg
Primary Mode of Elimination: Hepatic
Dosage Adjustments*

CrCl 50–80 mL/min	No change
CrCl 10–50 mL/min	No change
CrCl < 10 mL/min	No change
Post–HD dose	None
Post–PD dose	None
CVVH dose	None
Moderate hepatic insufficiency	No change
Severe hepatic insufficiency	No change; use caution

Antiretroviral Dosage Adjustments:

Atazanavir	Ritonavir 100 mg q24h + atazanavir 300 mg q24h with food
Delavirdine	Delavirdine: no change; ritonavir: No information
Efavirenz	Ritonavir 600 mg q12h (500 mg q12h for intolerance)
Indinavir	Ritonavir 100-200 mg q12h + indinavir 800 mg q12h, or 400 mg q12h of each drug
Nelfinavir	Ritonavir 400 mg q12h + nelfinavir 500-750 mg q12h
Nevirapine	No changes
Saquinavir	Ritonavir 400 mg q12h + saquinavir 400 mg q12h
Ketoconazole	Caution; do not exceed ketoconazole 200 mg q24h
Rifampin	Avoid
Rifabutin	Rifabutin 150 mg q48h or 3x/week

Drug Interactions: Antiretrovirals, rifabutin, rifampin (see dose adjustment grid, above); alprazolam, diazepam, estazolam, flurazepam, midazolam, triazolam, zolpidem, meperidine, propoxyphene, piroxicam, quinidine,

"Usual dose" assumes normal renal/hepatic function. * For renal insufficiency, give usual dose x 1 followed by maintenance dose per CrCl. For dialysis patients, dose the same as for CrCl < 10 mL/min and give supplemental (post-HD/PD dose) immediately after dialysis. CrCl = creatinine clearance; CVVH = continuous veno-venous hemofiltration; HD/PD = hemodialysis/peritoneal dialysis. See pp. 147-150 for explanations, p. 3 for abbreviations

amiodarone, encainide, flecainide, propafenone, astemizole, bepridil, bupropion, cisapride, clorazepate, clozapine, pimozide, St. John's wort, terfenadine (avoid); alfentanil, fentanyl, hydrocodone, tramadol, disopyramide, lidocaine, mexiletine, erythromycin, clarithromycin, warfarin, dronabinol, ondansetron, metoprolol, pindolol, propranolol, timolol, amlodipine, diltiazem, felodipine, isradipine, nicardipine, nifedipine, nimodipine, nisoldipine, nitrendipine, verapamil, etoposide, paclitaxel, tamoxifen, vinblastine, vincristine, loratadine, tricyclic antidepressants, paroxetine, nefazodone, sertraline, trazodone, fluoxetine, venlafaxine, fluvoxamine, cyclosporine, tacrolimus, chlorpromazine, haloperidol, perphenazine, risperidone, thioridazine, clozapine, pimozide, methamphetamine (↑ interacting drug levels); voriconazole (↓ voriconazole levels); telithromycin (↑ ritonavir levels); codeine, hydromorphone, methadone, morphine, ketoprofen, ketorolac, naproxen, diphenoxylate, oral contraceptives, theophylline (↓ interacting drug levels); carbamazepine, phenytoin, phenobarbital, clonazepam, dexamethasone, prednisone (↓ ritonavir levels, ↑ interacting drug levels; monitor anticonvulsant levels); metronidazole (disulfiram-like reaction); tenofovir, tobacco (↓ ritonavir levels); sildenafil (do not exceed 25 mg in 48 hrs); tadalafil (max. 10 mg/72 hrs); vardenafil (max. 2.5 mg/72 hrs)
Adverse Effects: Anorexia, anemia, leukopenia, hyperglycemia (including worsening diabetes, new-onset diabetes, DKA), h cholesterol/triglycerides (evaluate risk for coronary disease/pancreatitis), fat redistribution, ↑ CPK, nausea, vomiting, diarrhea, abdominal pain, circumoral/extremity paresthesias, ↑ SGOT/SGPT, pancreatitis, taste perversion, possible increased bleeding in hemophilia
Allergic Potential: Low
Safety in Pregnancy: B
Comments: Usually used at low dose (100-200 mg/day) as pharmacokinetic "booster" of other PI's. GI intolerance decreases over time. Take with food if possible (serum levels increase 15%, fewer GI side effects). Dose escalation regimen: day 1-2 (300 mg q12h), day 3-5 (400 mg q12h), day 6-13 (500 mg q12h), day 14 (600 mg q12h). Separate dosing from ddI by 2 hours. Refrigerate capsules (not oral solution) if temperature to exceed 78°F
Cerebrospinal Fluid Penetration: < 10%

REFERENCES:

Cameron DW, Japour AJ, Xu Y, et al. Ritonavir and saquinavir combination therapy for the treatment of HIV infection. AIDS 13:213-224, 1999.

Deeks SG, Smith M, Holodniy M, et al. HIV-1 protease inhibitors: A review for clinicians. JAMA 277:145-53, 1997.

Kaul DR, Cinti SK, Carver PL, et al. HIV protease inhibitors: Advances in therapy and adverse reactions, including metabolic complications. Pharmacotherapy 19:281-98, 1999.

Lea AP, Faulds D. Ritonavir. Drugs 52:541-6, 1996.

McDonald CK, Kuritzkes DR. Human immunodeficiency virus type 1 protease inhibitors. Arch Intern Med 157:951-9, 1997.

Panel on Clinical Practices for Treatment of HIV Infection. Guidelines for the use of antiretroviral agents in HIV-infected adults and adolescents. Department of Health and Human Services. www.aidsinfo.nih.gov/guidelines/. Jan 29, 2008.

Piliero PJ. Interaction between ritonavir and statins. Am J Med 112:510-1, 2002.

Rathbun RC, Rossi DR. Low-dose ritonavir for protease inhibitor pharmacokinetic enhancement. Ann Pharmacother 36:702-6, 2002.

Shepp DH, Stevens RC. Ritonavir boosting of HIV protease inhibitors. Antibiotics for Clinicians 9:301-311, 2005.

Website: www.TreatHIV.com

Saquinavir (Invirase) SQV

Drug Class: Antiretroviral protease inhibitor
Usual Dose: 1000 mg (PO) q12h (see comments) with ritonavir 100 mg (PO) q12h, or 400 mg (PO) q12h with ritonavir 400 mg (PO) q12h
Pharmacokinetic Parameters:
Peak serum level: 0.07 mcg/mL
Bioavailability: hard-gel (4%)
Excreted unchanged (urine): 13%
Serum half-life (normal/ESRD): 13 hrs/no data
Plasma protein binding: 98%
Volume of distribution (V_d): 10 L/kg
Primary Mode of Elimination: Hepatic

Dosage Adjustments*

CrCl 50–80 mL/min	No change
CrCl 10–50 mL/min	No change
CrCl < 10 mL/min	No change
Post–HD dose	None
Post–PD dose	None
CVVH dose	No change
Moderate hepatic insufficiency	No change
Severe hepatic insufficiency	Use caution

Antiretroviral Dosage Adjustments:

Darunavir	Avoid
Delavirdine	No Information
Efavirenz	Avoid use as sole PI
Indinavir	No information
Lopinavir/ritonavir 3 capsules q12h	Saquinavir 500 mg q12h
Nelfinavir	Saquinavir 1 gm q12h or 1200 mg q12h
Nevirapine	No information
Ritonavir	Ritonavir 100 mg q12h + saquinavir 1 gm q12h
Rifampin	Contraindicated
Rifabutin	Avoid

Drug Interactions: Antiretrovirals, rifabutin, rifampin (see dose adjustment grid, above); astemizole, terfenadine, benzodiazepines, cisapride, ergotamine, statins, St. John's wort (avoid if possible); carbamazepine, phenytoin, phenobarbital, dexamethasone, prednisone (↓ saquinavir levels, ↑ interacting drug levels; monitor anticonvulsant levels); clarithromycin, erythromycin, telithromycin (↑ saquinavir and macrolide levels); grapefruit juice, itraconazole, voriconazole, ketoconazole (↑ saquinavir levels); sildenafil (do not give > 25 mg/48 hrs); tadalafil (max. 10 mg/72 hrs), vardenafil (max. 2.5 mg/72 hrs)

Adverse Effects: Anorexia, headache, anemia, leukopenia, hyperglycemia (including worsening diabetes, new-onset diabetes, DKA), ↑ cholesterol/triglycerides (evaluate risk for coronary disease/pancreatitis), ↑ SGOT/SGPT, hyperuricemia, fat redistribution, possible increased bleeding in hemophilia

Allergic Potential: Low

Safety in Pregnancy: B

Comments: Take with food. Avoid garlic supplements, which ↓ saquinavir levels ~ 50%. Boosted dose: 1 gm saquinavir/100 mg ritonavir (PO) q12h. Preferred formulation is 500 mg hard-gel capsule (Invirase 500). Soft-gel capsules (Fortovase) no longer available

Cerebrospinal Fluid Penetration: < 1%

REFERENCES:

Borck C. Garlic supplements and saquinavir. Clin Infect Dis 35:343, 2002.

Cameron DW, Japour AJ, Xu Y, et al. Ritonavir and saquinavir combination therapy for the treatment of HIV infection. AIDS 13:213-224, 1999.

Cardiello PF, van Heeswijk RP, Hassink EA, et al. Simplifying protease inhibitor therapy with once-daily dosing of saquinavir soft-gelatin capsules/ritonavir (1600/100 mg): HIVNAT 001.3 study. J Acquir Immune Defic Syndr 29:464-70, 2002.

Hsu A, Granneman GR, Cao G, et al. Pharmacokinetic interactions between two human immunodeficiency virus protease inhibitors, ritonavir and saquinavir. Clin Pharmacol Ther 63:453-64, 1998.

Murphy RL, Brun S, Hicks C, et al. ABT-378/ritonavir plus stavudine and lamivudine for the treatment of antiretroviral-naive adults with HIV-1 infection: 48-week results. AIDS 15:F1-9, 2001.

Noble S, Faulds D. Saquinavir: A review of its pharmacology and clinical potential in the management of HIV infection. Drugs 52:93-112, 1996.

Perry CM, Noble S. Saquinavir soft-gel capsule formation: A review of its use in patients with HIV infection. Drugs 55;461-86, 1998.

Panel on Clinical Practices for Treatment of HIV Infection. Guidelines for the use of antiretroviral agents in HIV-infected adults and adolescents. Department of Health and Human Services.

www.aidsinfo.nih.gov/guidelines/. Jan 29, 2008.
Vella S, Floridia M. Saquinavir: Clinical pharmacology and efficacy. Clin Pharmacokinet 34:189-201, 1998.
Website: www.fortovase.com

Stavudine (Zerit) d4t

Drug Class: Antiretroviral NRTI (nucleoside reverse transcriptase inhibitor)
Usual Dose: ≥ 60 kg: 40 mg (PO) q12h; < 60 kg: 30 mg (PO) q12h
Pharmacokinetic Parameters:
Peak serum level: 4.2 mcg/mL
Bioavailability: 86%
Excreted unchanged (urine): 40%
Serum half-life (normal/ESRD): 1.0/5.1 hrs
Plasma protein binding: 0%
Volume of distribution (V_d): 0.5 L/kg
Primary Mode of Elimination: Renal
Dosage Adjustments* ≥ 60 kg / [≤ 60 kg]

CrCl 50–80 mL/min	40 mg (PO) q12h [30 mg (PO) q12h]
CrCl 25–50 mL/min	20 mg (PO) q12h [15 mg (PO) q12h]
CrCl ~ 10-25 mL/min	20 mg (PO) q24h [15 mg (PO) q24h]
Post–HD dose	20 mg (PO) [15 mg (PO)]
Post–PD dose	No information
CVVH dose	20 mg (PO) q24h [15 mg (PO) q24h]
Moderate hepatic insufficiency	No change
Severe hepatic insufficiency	No change

Drug Interactions: Ribavirin (↓ stavudine efficacy, ↑ risk of lactic acidosis); zidovudine (↓ stavudine levels); dapsone, INH, other neurotoxic agents (↑ risk of neuropathy), didanosine (↑ risk of neuropathy, lactic acidosis)
Adverse Effects: Drug fever/rash, nausea, vomiting, GI upset, diarrhea, headache, insomnia, dose dependent peripheral neuropathy, myalgias, pancreatitis, ↑ SGOT/SGPT, ↑ cholesterol, facial fat pad wasting, lipodystrophy, thrombocytopenia, leukopenia, lactic acidosis with hepatic steatosis (rare, but potentially life-threatening toxicity with use of NRTI's)
Allergic Potential: Low
Safety in Pregnancy: C
Comments: Pancreatitis may be severe/fatal. Avoid coadministration with AZT or ddC. Decrease dose in patients with peripheral neuropathy to 20 mg (PO) q12h. Pregnant women may be at increased risk for lactic acidosis/liver damage when stavudine is used with didanosine (ddI)
Cerebrospinal Fluid Penetration: 30%

REFERENCES:

Berasconi E, Boubaker K, Junghans C, et al Abnormalities of body fat distribution in HIV-infected persons treated with antiretroviral drugs: The Swiss HIV Cohort Study. J Acquir Immune Defic Syndr 31:50-5, 2002.
Dudley MN, Graham KK, Kaul S, et al. Pharmacokinetics of stavudine in patients with AIDS and AIDS-related complex. J Infect Dis 166:480-5, 1992.
FDA notifications. FDA changes information for stavudine label. Aids Alert 17:67, 2002.
Joly V, Flandre P, Meiffredy V, et al. Efficacy of zidovudine compared to stavudine, both in combination with lamivudine and indinavir, in human immunodeficiency virus-infected nucleoside-experienced patients with no prior exposure to lamivudine, stavudine, or protease inhibitors (Novavir trial). Antimicrob Agents Chemother 46:1906-13, 2002.
Lea AP, Faulds D. Stavudine: A review of its pharmacodynamic and pharmacokinetic properties and clinical potential in HIV infection. Drugs 51:846-64, 1996.
Miller KD, Cameron M, Wood LV, et al. Lactic acidosis and hepatic steatosis associated with use of stavudine: Report of four cases. Ann Intern Med. 133:192-196, 2000.
Murphy RL, Brun S, Hicks C, et al. ABT-378/ritonavir plus stavudine and lamivudine for the treatment of antiretroviral-naive adults with HIV-1 infection: 48-week results. AIDS 15:F1-9, 2001.
Panel on Clinical Practices for Treatment of HIV Infection. Guidelines for the use of antiretroviral agents in HIV-infected adults and adolescents. Department of Health and Human Services.

"Usual dose" assumes normal renal/hepatic function. * For renal insufficiency, give usual dose x 1 followed by maintenance dose per CrCl. For dialysis patients, dose the same as for CrCl < 10 mL/min and give supplemental (post-HD/PD dose) immediately after dialysis. CrCl = creatinine clearance; CVVH = continuous veno-venous hemofiltration; HD/PD = hemodialysis/peritoneal dialysis. See pp. 147-150 for explanations, p. 3 for abbreviations

www.aidsinfo.nih.gov/guidelines/. Jan 29, 2008.
Website: www.zerit.com

Tenofovir disoproxil fumarate (Viread) TDF

Drug Class: Antiretroviral (nucleotide analogue)
Usual Dose: 300 mg (PO) q24h
Pharmacokinetic Parameters:
Peak serum level: 0.29 mcg/mL
Bioavailability: 25%/39% (fasting/high fat meal)
Excreted unchanged (urine): 32%
Serum half-life (normal/ESRD): 17 hrs/no data
Plasma protein binding: 0.7-7.2%
Volume of distribution (V_d): 1.3 L/kg
Primary Mode of Elimination: Renal
Dosage Adjustments*

CrCl ≥ 50 mL/min	No change
CrCl 30–49 mL/min	300 mg (PO) q48h
CrCl 10–29 mL/min	300 mg (PO) 2x/week
CrCl < 10 mL/min	No information
Post–HD dose	300 mg q7d or after 12 hours on HD
Post–PD dose	No information
CVVH dose	No information
Moderate hepatic insufficiency	No change
Severe hepatic insufficiency	No change

Drug Interactions: Didanosine (if possible, avoid concomitant didanosine due to impaired CD4 response and increased risk of virologic failure); valganciclovir (↑ tenofovir levels); atazanavir, lopinavir/ritonavir (↑ tenofovir levels)(↓ atazanavir levels; use atazanavir 300 mg/ritonavir 100 mg with tenofovir); no clinically significant interactions with lamivudine, efavirenz, methadone, oral contraceptives. Not a substrate/inhibitor of cytochrome P-450 enzymes

Adverse Effects: Mild nausea, vomiting, GI upset, asthenia, headache, diarrhea, lactic acidosis with hepatic steatosis (rare, but potentially life-threatening with NRTI's), renal tubular acidosis, ↓ bone density (clinical significance unknown)
Allergic Potential: Low
Safety in Pregnancy: B
Comments: Eliminated by glomerular filtration/tubular secretion. May be taken with or without food. If possible, avoid concomitant didanosine (see drug interactions)
Cerebrospinal Fluid Penetration: No data

REFERENCES:

Gallant JE, DeJesus D, Arribas JR, et al. Tenofovir DF, emtricitabine, and efavirenz vs. zidovudine, lamivudine, and efavirenz for HIV. N Engl J Med 354:251-60, 2006.
Gallant JE. Efficacy and safety of tenofovir DF vs stavudine in combination therapy in antiretroviral-naive patients: a 3-year randomized trial. JAMA 2004;292:191-201.
Gallant JE, Deresinski S. Tenofovir disoproxil fumarate. Clin Infect Dis 37:944-50, 2003.
Guidelines for the Use of Antiretroviral Agents for HIV-1-infected Adults and Adolescents: recommendations of the Panel on Clinical Practices for Treatment of HIV Infection; www.aidsinfo.gov/guidelines/, Jan 29, 2008.
Jullien V, Treluye JM, Rey E, et al. Population pharmacokinetics of tenofovir in human immunodeficiency virus-infected patients taking highly active antiretroviral therapy. Antimicrobial Agents and Chemotherapy 49:3361-3366, 2005.
Terrault NA. Treatment of recurrent hepatitis B infection in liver transplant recipients. Liver Transpl 8(Suppl 1):S74-81, 2002.
Thromson CA. Prodrug of tenofovir diphosphate approved for combination HIV therapy. Am J Health Syst Pharm 59:18, 2002.
Website: www.viread.com

Tipranavir (Aptivus) TPV

Drug Class: Protease inhibitor
Usual Dose: 500 mg (PO) with ritonavir 200 mg (PO) q12h
Pharmacokinetic Parameters:
Peak serum level: 77-94 mcg/mL
Bioavailability: No data
Excreted unchanged (urine): 44%

"Usual dose" assumes normal renal/hepatic function. * For renal insufficiency, give usual dose x 1 followed by maintenance dose per CrCl. For dialysis patients, dose the same as for CrCl < 10 mL/min and give supplemental (post-HD/PD dose) immediately after dialysis. CrCl = creatinine clearance; CVVH = continuous veno-venous hemofiltration; HD/PD = hemodialysis/peritoneal dialysis. See pp. 147-150 for explanations, p. 3 for abbreviations

Serum half-life (normal/ESRD): 5.5-6/5.5-6 hrs
Plasma protein binding: 99.9%
Volume of distribution (V_d): 7-10 L/kg
Primary Mode of Elimination: Hepatic
Dosage Adjustments*

CrCl 50–80 mL/min	No change
CrCl 10–50 mL/min	No change
CrCl < 10 mL/min	No change
Post–HD dose	No change
Post–PD dose	No change
CVVH dose	No change
Mild hepatic insufficiency	No change
Moderate or severe hepatic insufficiency	Avoid

Drug Interactions: Rifabutin (↑ levels), clarithromycin (↑ levels), loperamide (↓ levels), statins (↑ risk of myopathy); abacavir, saquinavir, tenofovir, zidovudine, amprenavir/RTV, lopinavir/RTV (↓ levels). Aluminum/magnesium antacids (↓ absorption 25-30%). Ritonavir (↑ risk of hepatitis). St. John's Wort (↓ tipranavir levels). Keep refrigerated 2-8° C. Metabolized via CYP 3A4
Adverse Effects: Contraindicated in moderate/severe hepatic insufficiency. ↑ risk of hepatotoxicity in HIV patients co-infected with HBV/HCV. Case reports of intracerebral hemorrhage—use with caution in patients with coagulopathies
Allergic Potential: High. Tipranavir is a sulfonamide; use with caution in patients with sulfonamide allergies
Safety in Pregnancy: C
Comments: Should be taken with food. Increased bioavailability when taken with meals. Must be co-administered with 200 mg ritonavir. Tipranavir contains a sulfonamide moiety (as do darunavir and fosamprenavir)
Cerebrospinal Fluid Penetration: No data

REFERENCES:

Barbaro G, Scozzafava A, Mastrolorenzo A, et al. Highly active antiretroviral therapy: current state of the art, new agents and their pharmacological interactions useful for improving therapeutic outcome. Curr Pharm Des 11:1805-43, 2005.
Clotet B. Strategies for overcoming resistance in HIV-1 infected patients receiving HAART. AIDS Rev 6:123-30, 2004.
Croom KF, Keam SJ. Tipranavir: a ritonavir-boosted protease inhibitor. Drugs 65:1669-79, 2005.
de Mendoza C, Soriano V. Resistance to HIV protease inhibitors: mechanisms and clinical consequences. Curr Drug Metab 5:321-8, 2004.
Gulick RM. New antiretroviral drugs. Clin Microbiol Infect 9:186-93, 2003.
Hicks CB, Cahn P, Cooper DA, et al. Durable efficacy of tipranavir-ritonavir in combination with an optimised background regimen of antiretroviral drugs for treatment-experienced HIV-1-infected patients at 48 weeks in the Randomized Evaluation of Strategic Intervention in multi-drug reSistant patients with Tipranavir (RESIST) studies: an analysis of combined data from two randomized open-label trials. Lancet 368:466-75, 2006.
Kandula VR, Khanlou H, Farthing C. Tipranavir: a novel second-generation nonpeptidic protease inhibitor. Expert Rev Anti Infect Ther 3:9-21, 2005.
Kashuba AD. Drug-drug interactions and the pharmacotherapy of HIV infection. Top HIV Med 13:64-9, 2005.
Panel on Clinical Practices for Treatment of HIV Infection. Guidelines for the Use of Antiretroviral Agents in HIV-Infected Adults and Adolescents. Department of Health and Human Services. www.aidsinfo.nih.gov/guidelines/. Jan 29, 2008.
Plosker GL, Figgitt DP. Tripanavir. Drugs 63:1611-8, 2003.
Turner D, Schapiro JM,Brenner BG, Wainberg MA. The influence of protease inhibitor profiles on selection of HIV therapy in treatment-naïve patients. Antivir Ther 9:301-14, 2004.
Yeni P. Tipranovir: a protease inhibitor from a new class with distinct antiviral activity.
J Acquir Immune Defic Syndr 34 (Suppl 1):S91-4, 2003.
Website: www.aptivus.com

Zidovudine (Retrovir) ZDV Azidothymidine AZT

Drug Class: Antiretroviral NRTI (nucleoside reverse transcriptase inhibitor)
Usual Dose: 300 mg (PO) q12h (see comments). IV solution 10 mg/mL (dose 1 mg/kg 5-6 x/day)

"Usual dose" assumes normal renal/hepatic function. * For renal insufficiency, give usual dose x 1 followed by maintenance dose per CrCl. For dialysis patients, dose the same as for CrCl < 10 mL/min and give supplemental (post-HD/PD dose) immediately after dialysis. CrCl = creatinine clearance; CVVH = continuous veno-venous hemofiltration; HD/PD = hemodialysis/peritoneal dialysis. See pp. 147-150 for explanations, p. 3 for abbreviations

Pharmacokinetic Parameters:
Peak serum level: 1.2 mcg/mL
Bioavailability: 64%
Excreted unchanged (urine): 16%
Serum half-life (normal/ESRD): 1.1/1.4 hrs
Plasma protein binding: < 38%
Volume of distribution (V_d): 1.6 L/kg
Primary Mode of Elimination: Hepatic
Dosage Adjustments*

CrCl 50–80 mL/min	No change
CrCl 10–50 mL/min	No change
CrCl < 10 mL/min	300 mg (PO) q24h
HD/PD	100 mg (PO) q6-8h
Post–HD/PD dose	None
CVVH dose	300 mg (PO) q24h
Moderate or severe hepatic insufficiency	No information

Drug Interactions: Acetaminophen, atovaquone, fluconazole, methadone, probenecid, valproic acid (↑ zidovudine levels); clarithromycin, nelfinavir, rifampin, rifabutin (↓ zidovudine levels); dapsone, flucytosine, ganciclovir, interferon alpha, bone marrow suppressive/cytotoxic agents (↑ risk of hematologic toxicity); indomethacin (↑ levels of zidovudine toxic metabolite); phenytoin (↑ zidovudine levels, ↑ or ↓ phenytoin levels); ribavirin (↓ zidovudine effect; avoid)
Adverse Effects: Nausea, vomiting, GI upset, diarrhea, malaise, anorexia, leukopenia, severe anemia, macrocytosis, thrombocytopenia, headaches, ↑ SGOT/SGPT, hepatotoxicity, myalgias, myositis, symptomatic myopathy, insomnia, blue/black nail discoloration, asthenia, lactic acidosis with hepatic steatosis (rare, but potentially life-threatening toxicity with use of NRTI's)
Allergic Potential: Low
Safety in Pregnancy: C
Comments: Antagonized by ganciclovir or ribavirin. Also a component of Combivir and Trizivir. Patients on IV therapy should be switched to PO as soon as able to take oral medication. For IV administration, dilute in D5W to a concentration no greater than 4 mg/mL and infuse over 1 hour
Cerebrospinal Fluid Penetration: 60%

REFERENCES:

Barry M, Mulcahy F, Merry C, et al. Pharmacokinetics and potential interactions amongst antiretroviral agents used to treat patients with HIV infection. Clin Pharmacol 36:289-304, 1999.
Been-Tiktak AM, Boucher CA, Brun-Vezinet F, et al. Efficacy and safety of combination therapy with delavirdine and zidovudine: A European/Australian phase II trial. Intern J Antimcrob Agents 11:13-21, 1999.
McDowell JA, Lou Y, Symonds WS, et al. Multiple-dose pharmacokinetics and pharmacodynamics of abacavir alone and in combination with zidovudine in human immunodeficiency virus-infected adults. Antimicrob Agents Chemother 44:2061-7, 2000.
Montaner JS, Reiss P, Cooper D, et al. A randomized, double-blind trial comparing combinations of nevirapine, didanosine, and zidovudine for HIV-infected patients: The INCAS trial. Italy, the Netherlands, Canada and Australia Study. J Am Med Assoc 279:930-937, 1998.
Panel on Clinical Practices for Treatment of HIV Infection. Guidelines for the use of antiretroviral agents in HIV-infected adults and adolescents. Department of Health and Human Services. www.aidsinfo.nih.gov/guidelines/. Jan 29, 2008.
Piscitelli SC, Gallicano KD. Interactions among drugs for HIV and opportunistic infections. N Engl J Med 344:984-996, 2001.
Simpson DM. Human immunodeficiency virus-associated dementia: A review of pathogenesis, prophylaxis, and treatment studies of zidovudine therapy. Clin Infect Dis 29:19-34, 1999.
Website: www.TreatHIV.com

"Usual dose" assumes normal renal/hepatic function. * For renal insufficiency, give usual dose x 1 followed by maintenance dose per CrCl. For dialysis patients, dose the same as for CrCl < 10 mL/min and give supplemental (post-HD/PD dose) immediately after dialysis. CrCl = creatinine clearance; CVVH = continuous veno-venous hemofiltration; HD/PD = hemodialysis/peritoneal dialysis. See pp. 147-150 for explanations, p. 3 for abbreviations

MUTATIONS IN THE REVERSE TRANSCRIPTASE GENE ASSOCIATED WITH RESISTANCE TO REVERSE TRANSCRIPTASE INHIBITORS

Nucleoside and Nucleotide Reverse Transcriptase Inhibitors (nRTIs)[1]

Multi-nRTI Resistance: 69 Insertion Complex[2] (affects all nRTIs currently approved by the US FDA)

	M	A	▼	K	L	T	K
	41	62	69	70	210	215	219
	L	V	Insert	R	W	Y F	Q E

Multi-nRTI Resistance: 151 Complex[3] (affects all nRTIs currently approved by the US FDA except tenofovir)

	A	V	F	F	Q
	62	75	77	116	151
	V	I	L	Y	M

Multi-nRTI Resistance: Thymidine Analogue-associated Mutations[4,5] (TAMs; affects all nRTIs currently approved by the US FDA)

M	D	K	L	T	K
41	67	70	210	215	219
L	N	R	W	Y F	Q E

	K	L	Y	M
Abacavir[6]	65	74	115	184
	R	V	F	V

	K	L
Didanosine[7,8]	65	74
	R	V

	K	M
Emtricitabine	65	184
	R	V I

	K	M
Lamivudine	65	184
	R	V I

	M	D	K	L	T	K
Stavudine[4,5,9,10]	41	67	70	210	215	219
	L	N	R	W	Y F	Q E

	K	K
Tenofovir[11]	65	70
	R	R

	M	D	K	L	T	K
Zidovudine[4,5,9,10]	41	67	70	210	215	219
	L	N	R	W	Y F	Q E

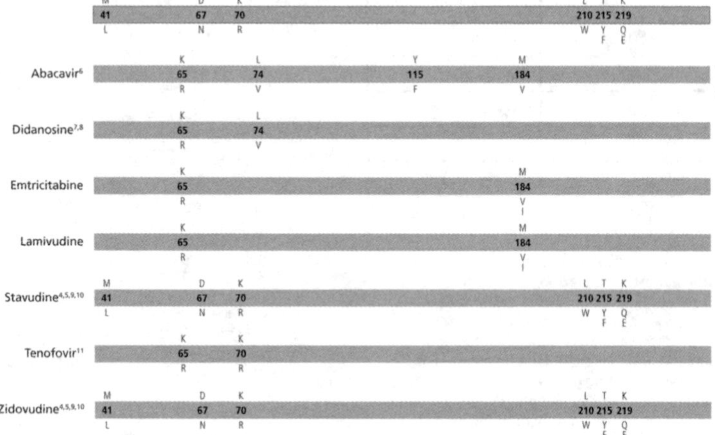

Nonnucleoside Reverse Transcriptase Inhibitors (NNRTIs)[1,12]

	L	K	V	V	Y	Y	G	P
Efavirenz	100	103	106	108	181	188	190	225
	I	N	M	I	C I	L	S A	H

	V	A	L	K	V	V	Y	G
Etravirine[13] (expanded access)	90	98	100	101	106	179	181	190
	I	G	I	E P	I	D F	C I V	S A

	L	K	V	V	Y	Y	G
Nevirapine	100	103	106	108	181	188	190
	I	N	A M	I	C I	C L H	A

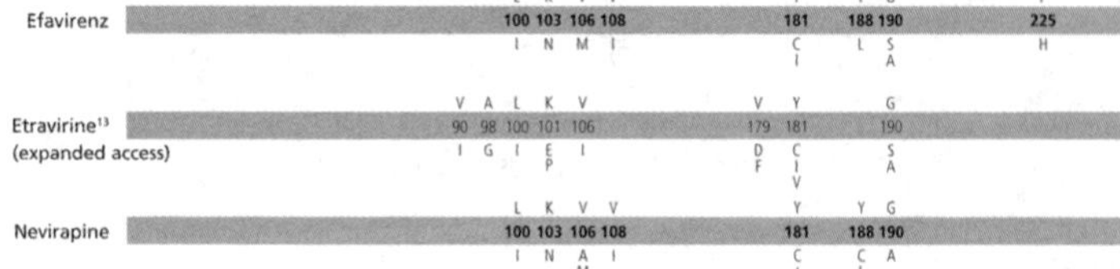

From: The International AIDS Society-USA (IAS-USA) Drug Resistance Mutations Group. Update of the Drug Resistance Mutations in HIV-1: 2007. Top HIV Med 2007;15(4):119-125. Reproduced with permission.

MUTATIONS IN THE PROTEASE GENE ASSOCIATED WITH RESISTANCE TO PROTEASE INHIBITORS[14,15,16,17]

Atazanavir +/– ritonavir[18]

Wild-type	L	G	K	L	V	L	E	M	M	G	I	F	I	D	I	I	A	G	V	I	I	N	L	I
Position	10	16	20	24	32	33	34	36	46	48	**50**	53	54	60	62	64	71	73	82	**84**	85	**88**	90	93
Substitution	I F V C	E	R M I T V	I	I	I F V	Q	I L V	I L	V	L	L Y	L V M T A	E	V	L M V	V I T L	C S T A	A T F I	V	V	S	M	L M

Fosamprenavir/ ritonavir

Wild-type	L	V	M	I	I	I	G	L	V	I	L
Position	10	32	46	47	**50**	54	73	76	82	**84**	90
Substitution	F I R V	I	I L	V	V	L V M	S	V	A F S T	V	M

Darunavir/ ritonavir[19]

Wild-type	V	V	L	I	I	I	G	L	I	L
Position	11	32	33	47	**50**	**54**	73	**76**	**84**	89
Substitution	I	I	F	V	V	M L	S	V	V	V

Indinavir/ ritonavir[20]

Wild-type	L	K	L	V	M	M	I	A	G	L	V	V	I	L
Position	10	20	24	32	36	**46**	54	71	73	76	77	**82**	**84**	90
Substitution	I R V	M R	I	I	I	I L	V	V T	S A	V	I	A F T	V	M

Lopinavir/ ritonavir[21]

Wild-type	L	K	L	V	L	M	I	I	F	I	L	A	G	L	V	I	L
Position	10	20	24	**32**	33	46	**47**	50	53	54	63	71	73	76	**82**	84	90
Substitution	F I R V	M R	I	I	F	I L	V A	V	L	V L A M T S	P	V T	S	V	A F T S	V	M

Nelfinavir[20,22]

Wild-type	L	D	M	M	A	V	V	I	N	L
Position	10	**30**	36	46	71	77	82	84	88	**90**
Substitution	F I	N	I	I L	V T	I	A F T S	V	D S	M

Saquinavir/ ritonavir

Wild-type	L	L	G	I	I	A	G	V	V	I	L
Position	10	24	**48**	54	62	71	73	77	82	84	**90**
Substitution	I R V	I	V	V L	V	V T	S	I	A F T S	V	M

Tipranavir/ ritonavir[23]

Wild-type	L	I	K	L	E	M	K	M	I	I	Q	H	T	V	N	I	L
Position	10	13	20	**33**	35	36	43	46	47	54	58	69	74	**82**	83	**84**	90
Substitution	V	V	M R	F	G	I	T	L	V	A M V	E	K	P	L T	D	V	M

MUTATIONS IN THE ENVELOPE GENE ASSOCIATED WITH RESISTANCE TO ENTRY INHIBITORS

Enfuvirtide[24]

Wild-type	G	I	V	Q	Q	N	N
Position	36	37	38	39	40	42	43
Substitution	D S	V	A M E	R	H	T	D

Maraviroc[25]: See User Note

MUTATIONS IN THE INTEGRASE GENE ASSOCIATED WITH RESISTANCE TO INTEGRASE INHIBITORS

Raltegravir[26] (expanded access)

Wild-type	Q	N
Position	**148**	**155**
Substitution	H K R	H

MUTATIONS

[Legend labels:] Insertion; Amino acid, wild-type — L; Amino acid position — Major (boldface type; protease only)[15] — **90**; Amino acid substitution conferring resistance — M; Minor (lightface type; protease only)[15] — 54

Amino acid abbreviations: A, alanine; C, cysteine; D, aspartate; E, glutamate; F, phenylalanine; G, glycine; H, histidine; I, isoleucine; K, lysine; L, leucine; M, methionine; N, asparagine; P, proline; Q, glutamine; R, arginine; S, serine; T, threonine; V, valine; W, tryptophan; Y, tyrosine.

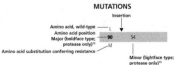

The International AIDS Society–USA Drug Resistance Mutations Group reviews new data on HIV drug resistance in order to maintain a current list of mutations associated with clinical resistance to HIV. This list includes mutations that may contribute to a reduced virologic response to a drug.

The mutations listed have been identified by 1 or more of the following criteria: (1) in vitro passage experiments or validation of contribution to resistance by using site-directed mutagenesis; (2) susceptibility testing of laboratory or clinical isolates; (3) genetic sequencing of viruses from patients in whom the drug is failing; (4) correlation studies between genotype at baseline and virologic response in patients exposed to the drug. In addition, the group only reviews data that have been published or have been presented at a scientific conference. Drugs that have been approved by the US Food and Drug Administration (FDA) as well as drugs available in expanded access programs are included (listed in alphabetic order by drug class). User notes provide additional information as necessary. Although the Drug Resistance Mutations Group works to maintain a complete and current list of these mutations, it cannot be assumed that the list presented here is exhaustive. Readers are encouraged to consult the literature and experts in the field for clarification or more information about specific mutations and their clinical impact.

User Notes

1. Numerous nucleoside (or nucleotide) reverse transcriptase inhibitor (nRTI) mutations, such as the M41L, L210W, and T215Y mutations, may lead to viral hypersusceptibility to the nonnucleoside reverse transcriptase inhibitors (NNRTIs) in nRTI-treated individuals. The presence of these mutations may improve subsequent virologic response to NNRTI-containing regimens in NNRTI treatment-naive individuals (Shulman et al, *AIDS*, 2004; Haubrich et al, *AIDS*, 2002; Tozzi, *J Infect Dis*, 2004; Katzenstein et al, *AIDS*, 2003). NNRTI hypersusceptibility can be conferred by 2 distinct phenotypes: increased enzyme susceptibility to NNRTI (eg, V118I/T215Y) or decreased virion associated levels of reverse transcriptase (eg, H208Y/T215Y and V118I/H208Y/T215Y). The viruses that contained less reverse transcriptase replicated less efficiently than those with wild-type levels of reverse transcriptase. (Clark et al, *Antivir Ther*, 2006). The clinical relevance of all these mutations has not been assessed.

2. The 69 insertion complex consists of a substitution at codon 69 (typically T69S) and an insertion of 2 or more amino acids (S-S, S-A, S-G, or others). The 69 insertion complex is associated with resistance to all nRTIs currently approved by the US FDA when present with 1 or more thymidine analogue-associated mutations (TAMs) at codons 41, 210, or 215 (Miller et al, *J Infect Dis*, 2004). Some other amino acid changes from the wild-type T at codon 69 without the insertion may also be associated with broad nRTI resistance.

3. Tenofovir retains activity against the Q151M complex of mutations (Miller et al, *J Infect Dis*, 2004).

4. Multi-nRTI resistance mutations, also known as nucleoside analogue-associated mutations (NAMs), are associated with resistance to numerous nRTIs. The M41L, D67N, K70R, L210W, T215Y/F, and K219Q/E are known as TAMs. TAMs are a subset of NAMs that are selected by the thymidine analogues zidovudine and stavudine and are associated with cross-resistance to all nRTIs currently approved by the US FDA (Larder et al, *Science*, 1989; Kellam et al, *Proc Natl Acad Sci USA*, 1992; Calvez et al, *Antivir Ther*, 2002; Kuritzkes et al, *J Acquir Immune Defic Syndr*, 2004). Mutations at the C-terminal reverse transcriptase domains (amino acids 293–560) outside of regions depicted on the figure bars may prove to be important for HIV drug resistance. Mutations in the connection (A371V) and RNase H (Q509L) domains of reverse transcriptase are coselected on the same genome as TAMs and increase significantly zidovudine resistance when combined with TAMs. They also increase, although to a much lesser extent, cross-resistance to lamivudine, abacavir, and tenofovir but not to stavudine or didanosine (Brehm et al, *Antivir Ther*, 2006). When the polymerase domain contains TAMs, mutations in the connection domain (E312Q, G335C/D, N348I, A360I/V, V365I, and A376S) increase resistance to zidovudine from 11-fold to as much as 536-fold over wild-type reverse transcriptase (Nikolenko et al, *Proc Natl Acad Sci USA*, 2007). Three mutations (N348I, T369I, and E399D) in the reverse transcriptase C-terminus are associated with the increased resistance to zidovudine and to NNRTIs. Mutations at this level could modulate NNRTI resistance by affecting dimerization of p66/p51 heterodimers (Gupta et al, *Antivir Ther*, 2006). Since the clinical relevance of these mutations has not been demonstrated, they are not depicted on the figure bars.

5. The E44D and the V118I mutations increase the level of resistance to zidovudine and stavudine in the setting of TAMs, and correspondingly increase cross-resistance to the other nRTIs. The significance of E44D or V118I when each occurs in isolation is unknown (Romano et al, *J Infect Dis*, 2002; Walter et al, *Antimicrob Agents Chemother*, 2002; Girouard et al, *Antivir Ther*, 2002).

6. The M184V mutation alone does not appear to be associated with a reduced virologic response to abacavir in vivo (Harrigan et al, *J Infect Dis*, 2000; Lanier et al, *Antivir Ther*, 2004). When present with 2 or 3 TAMs, M184V contributes to reduced susceptibility to abacavir and is associated with impaired virologic response in vivo (Lanier et al, *Antivir Ther*, 2004). The M184V plus 4 or more TAMs resulted in no virologic response to abacavir in vivo (Lanier et al, *Antivir Ther*, 2004).

7. The K65R mutation may be selected by didanosine and is associated in vitro with decreased susceptibility to the drug (Winters et al, *Antimicrob Agents Chemother*, 1997). The impact of the K65R mutation in vivo is unclear.

8. The presence of 3 of the following—M41L, D67N, L210W, T215Y/F, and K219Q/E—has been associated with resistance to didanosine (Marcelin et al, *Antimicrob Agents Chemother*, 2005). The K70R and M184V mutations are not associated with a decreased virologic response to didanosine in vivo (Molina et al, *J Infect Dis*, 2005).

9. The presence of the M184V mutation appears to delay or prevent emergence of TAMs (Kuritzkes et al, *AIDS*, 1996). This effect may be overcome by an accumulation of TAMs or other mutations. The clinical significance of this effect of M184V is not known.

10. The T215A/C/D/E/G/H/I/L/N/S/V substitutions are revertant mutations at codon 215, conferring increased risk of virologic failure of zidovudine or stavudine in antiretroviral-naive patients (Riva et al, *Antivir Ther*, 2002; Chappey et al, *Antivir Ther*, 2003; Violin et al, *AIDS*, 2004). In vitro studies and preliminary clinical studies suggest that the T215Y mutant may emerge quickly from one of these mutations in the presence of zidovudine or stavudine (Garcia-Lerma et al, *J Virol*, 2004; Lanier et al, *Antivir Ther*, 2002; Riva et al, *Antivir Ther*, 2002).

11. The K65R mutation is associated with a reduced virologic response to tenofovir in

vivo (Miller et al, *J Infect Dis*, 2004). A reduced response occurs in the presence of 3 or more TAMs inclusive of either M41L or L210W (Miller et al, *J Infect Dis*, 2004). Slightly increased treatment responses to tenofovir in vivo were observed if M184V was present (Miller et al, *J Infect Dis*, 2004).

12. The long-term virologic response to sequential NNRTI use is poor, particularly when 2 or more mutations are present (Antinori et al, *AIDS Res Hum Retroviruses*, 2002; Lecossier et al, *J Acquir Immune Defic Syndr*, 2005). The K103N or Y188L mutation alone prevents the clinical utility of all NNRTIs currently approved by the US FDA (Antinori et al, *AIDS Res Human Retroviruses*, 2002).The V106M mutation is more common in HIV-1 subtype C than in subtype B, and confers cross-resistance to all currently approved NNRTIs (Brenner et al, *AIDS*, 2003; Cane et al, *J Clin Micro*, 2001).

13. The impact of most mutations depends on the simultaneous presence of Y181C; Y181C has impact only when present with 1 or more of these mutations. Substantial virologic response was still seen in clinical trials despite the presence of single mutations (Vingerhoets et al, *Antivir Ther*, 2007).

14. The same mutations usually emerge whether or not PIs are boosted with low-dose ritonavir, although the relative frequency of mutations may differ. Data on the selection of mutations in antiretroviral-naive patients in whom a boosted PI is failing are very limited. Numerous mutations are often necessary to significantly impact virologic response to a boosted PI. Although numbers vary for the different drugs, 3 or more mutations are often required.

15. Resistance mutations in the protease gene are classified as either "major" or "minor," if data are available.

Major mutations in the protease gene are defined in general either as those selected first in the presence of the drug; or those shown at the biochemical or virologic level to lead to an alteration in drug binding or an inhibition of viral activity or viral replication. Major mutations have an effect on drug susceptibility phenotype. In general, these mutations tend to be the primary contact residues for drug binding.

Minor mutations generally emerge later than major mutations, and by themselves do not have a significant effect on phenotype. In some cases, their effect may be to improve replicative fitness of the virus containing major mutations. However, some minor mutations are present as common polymorphic changes in HIV-1nonsubtype B clades, such as K20I/R and M36I in protease.

16. Ritonavir is not listed separately as it is currently used at therapeutic doses as a pharmacologic booster of other PIs. At higher doses tested previously in humans, ritonavir administered as monotherapy produces mutations similar to those produced by indinavir (Molla, *Nature Med*, 1996).

17. HIV-1 Gag cleavage site changes can cause PI resistance in vitro. It has been observed that mutations in the N-terminal part of *gag* (MA: E40K; L75R; K113E and CA: M200I; A224A/V), outside the cleavage site, contribute directly to PI resistance by enhancing the overall Gag processing by wild-type protease. (Nijhuis et al, *PLoS Med*, 2007). The clinical relevance of these mutations has not been assessed.

18. In most patients in whom an atazanavir/ritonavir-containing regimen was failing virologically, accumulations of the following 13 mutations were found (L10F/I/V, G16E, L33F/I/V, M46I/L, I54L/V/M/T, D60E, I62V, A71I/T/L, V82A/T, I84V, I85V, L90M, and I93L). Seven mutations were retained in an atazanavir score (L10F/I/V, G16E, L33F/I/V, M46I/L, D60E, I84V, I85V); the presence of 3 or more of these mutations predicts a reduced virologic response at 3 months, particularly when L90M was present (Vora et al, *AIDS*, 2006; http://www.hivfrenchresistance.org/2006/tab2.html). A different report (Bertoli et al, *Antivir Ther*, 2006) found that the presence of 0, 1, 2, or greater than or equal to 3 of the following mutations were associated with 92%, 93%, 75%, and 0% virologic response to atazanavir/ritonavir: L10C/I/V, V32I, E34Q, M46I/L, F53L, I54A/M/V, V82A/F/I/T, I84V; presence of I15E/G/L/V, H69K/M/N/Q/R/T/Y, and I72M/T/V improved the chances of response. For unboosted atazanavir, the presence of 0, 1, 2, or greater than or equal to 3 of the following mutations was associated with 83%, 67%, 6%, and 0% response rates: G16E, V32I, K20I/M/R/T/V, L33F/I/V, F53L/Y, I64L/M/V, A71I/T/V, I85V, I93L/M.

19. Darunavir (formerly TMC-114), boosted with ritonavir, was approved by the US FDA in June 2006. Resistance data are therefore still preliminary and limited. HIV RNA response to boosted darunavir correlated with baseline susceptibility and the presence of multiple specific PI mutations. Reductions in response were associated with increasing numbers of the mutations indicated in the bar. Some of these mutations appear to have a greater effect on susceptibility than others (eg, I50V versus V11I). Further study and analysis in other populations are required to refine and validate these findings.

20. The mutations depicted on the chart bar cannot be considered to be comprehensive since little relevant research has been reported in recent years to update the resistance and cross-resistance patterns for this drug.

21. In PI-experienced patients, the accumulation of 6 or more of the mutations indicated on the bar is associated with a reduced virologic response to lopinavir/ritonavir (Masquelier et al, *Antimicrob Agents Chemother*, 2002; Kempf et al, *J Virol*, 2001). The product information states that accumulation of 7 or 8 mutations confers resistance to the drug. In contrast, in those in whom lopinavir/ritonavir is their first PI used, resistance to this drug at the time of virologic rebound is rare. However, there is emerging evidence that specific mutations, most notably I47A (and possibly I47V) and V32I are associated with high-level resistance (Mo et al, *J Virol*, 2005; Friend et al, *AIDS*, 2004; Kagan et al, *Protein Sci*, 2005).

22. In some nonsubtype-B HIV-1, D30N is selected less frequently than other PI mutations (Gonzalez et al, *Antivir Ther*, 2004).

23. Accumulation of more than 2 mutations at positions 33, 82, 84, and 90 correlate with reduced virologic response to tipranavir/ritonavir, although an independent role for L90M was not found. Detailed analyses of data from phase II and III trials in PI-experienced patients identified mutations associated with reduced susceptibility or virologic response. These include: L10V, I13V, K20M/R, L33F, E35G, M36I, K43T, M46L, I47V, I54A/M/V, Q58E, H69K, T74P, V82L/T, N83D, and I84V. Accumulation of these mutations is associated with reduced response. Subsequent genotype-phenotype and genotype-virologic response analyses determined some mutations have a greater effect than others (eg, I84V versus I54M). Refinement and clinical validation of these findings are pending (Schapiro et al, CROI, 2005; Mayers et al, *Antivir Ther*, 2004; Hall et al, *Antivir Ther*, 2003; McCallister et al, *Antivir Ther*, 2003; Parkin et al, CROI, 2006; Bacheler et al, European HIV Drug Resistance Workshop, 2006).

24. Although resistance to enfuvirtide is associated primarily with mutations in the first heptad repeat (HR1) region of the gp41 envelope gene, wild-type viruses in the

depicted HR1 region vary 500-fold in susceptibility. Such pretreatment susceptibility differences were not associated with differences in clinical responses (Labrosse et al, *J Virol*, 2003). Furthermore, mutations or polymorphisms in other regions in the envelope (eg, the HR2 region or those yet to be identified) as well as coreceptor usage and density may affect susceptibility to enfuvirtide (Reeves et al, *Proc Natl Acad Sci USA*, 2002; Reeves et al, *J Virol*, 2004; Xu et al, *Antimicrob Agents Chemother*, 2005). Thus, testing to detect only the depicted HR1 mutations may not be adequate for clinical management of suspected failure (Reeves et al, *J Virol*, 2004; Menzo et al, *Antimicrob Agents Chemother*, 2004; Poveda et al, *J Med Virol*, 2004; Sista et al, *AIDS*, 2004; Su, *Antivir Ther*, 2004).

25. Maraviroc activity is limited to patients with only CCR5 (R5)-using virus detectable; CXCR4 (X4)-CCR5 mixed tropic viruses and X4-using viruses do not respond to maraviroc treatment. Some cases of virologic failure during maraviroc therapy are associated with outgrowth of X4 virus that preexists as a minority population below the level of assay detection. Mutations in the HIV-1 gp120 molecule that allow the virus to bind to R5 receptors in the presence of drug have been described in viruses from some patients whose virus remained R5 at the time of virologic failure. A number of such mutations have been identified, and the phenotypic manifestation of this drug resistance is a reduction in the maximal percentage inhibition (MPI) rather than the increase in the 50% inhibitory concentration (IC_{50}; defined by fold increase) that is characteristic of resistance to other classes of antiretrovirals. The resistance profile for maraviroc is too complex to be depicted on the figures. The frequency and rate at which maraviroc resistance mutations emerge are not yet known.

26. Raltegravir failure was associated with integrase mutations in 2 distinct genetic pathways defined by 2 or more mutations including: (1) a signature (major) mutation at either Q148H/K/R or N155H; and (2) 1 or more minor mutations unique to each pathway. Minor mutations described in the Q148H/K/R pathway include L74M + E138A, E138K, or G140S. The most common mutation pattern in this pathway is Q148H + G140S; this Q148H + G140S pattern exhibits the greatest loss of drug susceptibility. Mutations described in the N155H pathway include this primary mutation plus either L74M, E92Q, T97A, E92Q + T97A, Y143H, G163K/R, V151I, or D232N (Hazuda et al, *Antivir Ther*, 2007).

SELECTED KEY INTERNET RESOURCES

- AIDSinfo - A Service of the Department of Health and Human Services (www.aidsinfo.nih.gov)
- International AIDS Society - USA (www.iasusa.org)
- Comprehensive HIV/AIDS Resource (www.thebody.com)
- National AIDS Treatment Advocacy Project (www.natap.org)
- National Institute of Allergy and Infectious Diseases (niaid.nih.gov/daids/aids.html)
- National Library of Medicine - AIDS Portal (sis.nlm.nih.gov/hiv.html)
- National Library of Medicine - MedlinePlus AIDS page (www.nlm.nih.gov/medlineplus/)
- HIV/HCV Co-infection Center of Excellence (www.uchsc.edu/mpaetc/coinfection)
- Chronic Hepatitis C: Current Disease Management (www.niddk.nig.gov/)
- Hep C Connection (www.hepc-connection.org)
- Hepatitis Resource Network (HRN) (www.h-r-n.org)
- HIV and Hepatitis.com (www.hivandhepatitis.com)
- Johns Hopkins Hepatitis C and HIV Coinfection Information (www.hopkins-hepc.org)
- Management of Hepatitis C: 2002, NIH Consensus Statement: (http://consensus.nih.gov/cons/cons.htm)
- National HIV/AIDS Clinicians' Consultation Center (www.ucsf.ed/hivcntr)
- The National AIDS Treatment Advocacy Project (www.natap.org)
- National Clinicians' Postexposure Prophylaxis Hotline (www.ucsf.edu/hivcntr)
- HIV Drug Interactions: www.HIV-druginteractions.org

INDEX

ORDERING INFORMATION — HIV ESSENTIALS

Five Easy Ways to Order

Phone: 1-800-832-0034
Fax: 978-443-8000
E-mail: info@jbpub.com
Internet (faster service): www.jbpub.com

Mail: Jones and Bartlett Publishers
40 Tall Pine Drive
Sudbury, MA 01776

Substantial discounts on bulk quantities of Jones and Bartlett's publications are available to corporations, professional associations, and other qualified organizations. For details and specific discount information, contact the special sales department at Jones and Bartlett via the above contact information or send an email to specialsales@jbpub.com.

PHYSICIANS' PRESS

A DIVISION OF JONES AND BARTLETT PUBLISHERS

Sudbury, Massachusetts

BOSTON TORONTO LONDON SINGAPORE